Welcome to the *Fit Men Cookbook*, your ultimate guide to quick, healthy, and flavorful meals designed specifically for the modern man on the go. In today's fast-paced world, maintaining a healthy lifestyle can often feel challenging, but it doesn't have to be. This cookbook is your passport to delicious, nutritious meals that fuel your body and support your active lifestyle.

Inside these pages, you'll discover over 110 recipes meticulously crafted to provide the perfect balance of taste, convenience, and nutrition. From energizing breakfasts to satisfying dinners and everything in between, each recipe is designed to be quick and easy to prepare, without compromising on flavor or quality.

Whether you're a fitness enthusiast, a busy professional, or someone looking to improve their eating habits, this cookbook is here to simplify your meal planning and inspire you to eat well. You'll find recipes that fit into your hectic schedule without sacrificing the nutrients your body needs to perform at its best.

Key features of the Fit Men Cookbook include:

- **Quick and Easy Recipes:** Meals that can be prepared in minimal time, perfect for busy days.

- **Healthy Ingredients:** Nutrient-dense recipes that support your fitness and wellness goals.

- **Flavorful Options:** Delicious dishes that prove eating healthy doesn't mean sacrificing taste.

- **Meal Prep Tips:** Strategies to streamline your cooking process and save time during the week.

- **Inspiring Photography:** Visuals that showcase the vibrant colors and textures of each dish, enticing you to dive into the kitchen.

Whether you're whipping up a post-workout protein-packed meal or planning ahead for a week of nutritious lunches, the *Fit Men Cookbook* is your partner in achieving and maintaining a balanced, healthy lifestyle. Let's embark on this culinary journey together and discover how easy and enjoyable healthy eating can be

1. Southwest Chicken Salad

Ingredient:

• 2 boneless, skinless chicken breasts
• 1 tsp chili powder
• 1 tsp cumin
• 1/2 tsp garlic powder
• Salt and pepper to taste
• 1 head romaine lettuce, chopped
• 1 cup cherry tomatoes, halved
• 1 avocado, diced
• 1/2 cup black beans, rinsed and drained
• 1/4 cup shredded cheddar cheese
• 2 tbsp chopped cilantro
• 2 tbsp lime juice
• 2 tbsp olive oil
• 1 tbsp honey
• 1 tsp Dijon mustard

Instructions:

1. Preheat your grill or grill pan to medium•high heat. Season the chicken breasts with chili powder, cumin, garlic powder, salt, and pepper.

2. Grill the chicken for 5•7 minutes per side, or until cooked through. Allow the chicken to rest for a few minutes, then slice or shred it.

3. In a large salad bowl, combine the chopped romaine lettuce, cherry tomatoes, avocado, black beans, shredded cheddar cheese, and chopped cilantro.

4. In a small bowl, whisk together the lime juice, olive oil, honey, and Dijon mustard to make the dressing.

5. Add the grilled chicken to the salad and drizzle the dressing over the top. Toss everything together until well combined.

6. Serve the Southwest Chicken Salad immediately and enjoy!

This salad is packed with protein, healthy fats, and a variety of fresh vegetables, making it a nutritious and satisfying meal for both men and women. The combination of spices, citrus, and creamy avocado creates a delicious and flavorful dish.

2. Spicy Garlic Shrimp with Quinoa

Ingredient:

- 1 cup uncooked quinoa, rinsed
- 2 cups low•sodium chicken or vegetable broth
- 1 lb large shrimp, peeled and deveined
- 3 cloves garlic, minced
- 1 tsp red pepper flakes (or more to taste)
- 2 tbsp olive oil
- 2 tbsp fresh lemon juice
- 2 tbsp chopped fresh parsley
- Salt and pepper to taste

Instructions:

1. In a medium saucepan, combine the quinoa and broth. Bring to a boil, then reduce heat to low, cover, and simmer for 15•20 minutes, or until the quinoa is tender and the liquid is absorbed. Fluff with a fork and set aside.

2. In a large skillet, heat the olive oil over medium•high heat. Add the minced garlic and red pepper flakes, and cook for 1 minute, stirring constantly, until fragrant.

3. Add the shrimp to the skillet and cook for 2•3 minutes per side, or until the shrimp are pink and opaque. Be careful not to overcook the shrimp.

4. Remove the skillet from the heat and stir in the lemon juice and chopped parsley. Season with salt and pepper to taste.

5. To serve, divide the cooked quinoa among plates or bowls, and top with the spicy garlic shrimp. Enjoy!

This dish is a great source of lean protein from the shrimp, complex carbohydrates from the quinoa, and healthy fats from the olive oil. The combination of spicy, garlicky flavors makes it a delicious and satisfying meal for both men and women.

3. Greek Chicken Bowls

Ingredient:

- 1 lb boneless, skinless chicken breasts
- 2 tbsp olive oil
- 2 tsp dried oregano
- 1 tsp garlic powder
- 1 tsp lemon zest
- Salt and pepper to taste
- 1 cup cooked quinoa or brown rice
- 1 cup chopped cucumber
- 1 cup cherry tomatoes, halved
- 1/2 cup crumbled feta cheese
- 1/4 cup sliced kalamata olives
- 2 tbsp chopped fresh parsley
- 2 tbsp lemon juice
- 1 tbsp red wine vinegar
- 1 tsp Dijon mustard

Instructions:

1. Preheat your oven to 400°F (200°C).

2. In a small bowl, combine the olive oil, oregano, garlic powder, lemon zest, salt, and pepper. Rub the seasoning mixture all over the chicken breasts.

3. Place the seasoned chicken on a baking sheet and roast in the preheated oven for 20•25 minutes, or until the chicken is cooked through and reaches an internal temperature of 165°F (75°C).

4. While the chicken is cooking, prepare the rest of the ingredients. In a large bowl, combine the cooked quinoa or brown rice, chopped cucumber, cherry tomatoes, crumbled feta cheese, sliced kalamata olives, and chopped parsley.

5. In a small bowl, whisk together the lemon juice, red wine vinegar, and Dijon mustard to make the dressing.

6. Once the chicken is cooked, slice or shred it and add it to the bowl with the other ingredients.

7. Drizzle the dressing over the chicken and vegetable mixture, and gently toss to combine. Serve the Greek Chicken Bowls immediately, and enjoy!

This dish is packed with lean protein from the chicken, complex carbohydrates from the quinoa or brown rice, and a variety of fresh vegetables and Mediterranean flavors. It's a nutritious and satisfying meal that can be enjoyed by both men and women.

4. Spaghetti Squash Lasagna

Ingredient:

- 1 tsp dried basil
- Salt and pepper to taste
- 1 cup part•skim ricotta cheese
- 1 egg
- 1/2 cup grated Parmesan cheese
- 1 cup shredded mozzarella cheese

- 1 medium spaghetti squash, halved lengthwise and seeds removed
- 1 lb ground turkey or lean ground beef
- 1 onion, diced
- 3 cloves garlic, minced
- 1 (28 oz) can crushed tomatoes
- 2 tsp dried oregano

Instructions:

1. Preheat your oven to 400ºF (200ºC). Place the spaghetti squash halves cut•side down on a baking sheet and roast for 30•40 minutes, or until tender when pierced with a fork. Allow the squash to cool slightly, then use a fork to shred the flesh into spaghetti•like strands.

2. In a large skillet, cook the ground turkey or beef over medium heat, breaking it up as it cooks, until no longer pink, about 5•7 minutes. Add the diced onion and minced garlic, and cook for an additional 2•3 minutes, until the onion is translucent.

3. Stir in the crushed tomatoes, dried oregano, and dried basil. Season with salt and pepper to taste. Simmer the sauce for 10•15 minutes, stirring occasionally, to allow the flavors to meld.

4. In a small bowl, mix together the ricotta cheese, egg, and 1/4 cup of the Parmesan cheese.

5. Grease a 9x13 inch baking dish. Layer half of the shredded spaghetti squash in the bottom of the dish. Top with the ricotta cheese mixture, followed by half of the meat sauce. Repeat the layers, ending with the meat sauce.

6. Sprinkle the remaining 1/4 cup Parmesan cheese and the 1 cup of shredded mozzarella cheese over the top.

7. Bake the lasagna for 25•30 minutes, or until the cheese is melted and bubbly.

8. Allow the lasagna to cool for 5•10 minutes before serving.

This Spaghetti Squash Lasagna is a healthier, low•carb alternative to traditional lasagna, but it still delivers on flavor and satisfaction. It's a great option for both men and women who are looking for a nutritious and delicious meal.

5. Beef & Veggie Stir·Fry

Ingredient:

- 1 lb beef sirloin or flank steak, thinly sliced
- 2 tbsp low·sodium soy sauce
- 1 tbsp rice vinegar
- 1 tsp sesame oil
- 1 tsp cornstarch
- 2 tbsp olive oil
- 3 cloves garlic, minced
- 1 inch piece fresh ginger, peeled and grated
- 1 red bell pepper, sliced
- 1 cup broccoli florets
- 1 cup snow peas or snap peas
- 1 cup sliced mushrooms
- 2 green onions, sliced
- Salt and pepper to taste
- Cooked brown rice or quinoa, for serving (optional)

Instructions:

1. In a medium bowl, combine the sliced beef, soy sauce, rice vinegar, sesame oil, and cornstarch. Toss to coat the beef and let it marinate for 15·20 minutes.

2. Heat the olive oil in a large skillet or wok over high heat. Add the minced garlic and grated ginger, and cook for 1 minute, stirring constantly, until fragrant.

3. Add the marinated beef to the skillet and stir·fry for 2·3 minutes, until the beef is lightly browned.

4. Add the sliced bell pepper, broccoli florets, snow peas or snap peas, and sliced mushrooms to the skillet. Stir·fry for an additional 3·5 minutes, until the vegetables are tender·crisp.

5. Remove the skillet from the heat and stir in the sliced green onions. Season the stir·fry with salt and pepper to taste.

6. Serve the Beef & Veggie Stir·Fry immediately, over a bed of cooked brown rice or quinoa, if desired.

This Beef & Veggie Stir·Fry is a nutritious and flavorful dish that can be enjoyed by both men and women. It's packed with lean protein, fiber·rich vegetables, and a savory, umami·rich sauce. The quick cooking time and versatile ingredients make it a great option for a healthy and satisfying meal.

8. BBQ Chicken Stuffed Sweet Potatoes

Ingredient:

- 4 medium sweet potatoes
- 1 lb boneless, skinless chicken breasts
- 1 cup barbecue sauce (use a sugar•free or low•sugar variety)
- 1/2 cup shredded cheddar cheese
- 2 tbsp chopped fresh cilantro (optional)

Instructions:

1. Preheat your oven to 400°F (200°C).

2. Pierce the sweet potatoes several times with a fork and place them directly on the oven rack. Bake for 45•60 minutes, or until they are tender when pierced with a fork.

3. While the sweet potatoes are baking, place the chicken breasts in a slow cooker or Instant Pot. Pour the barbecue sauce over the chicken and cook until the chicken is cooked through and shreds easily, about 3•4 hours on low in the slow cooker or 15•20 minutes on high pressure in the Instant Pot.

4. Once the sweet potatoes are cooked, remove them from the oven and let them cool slightly. Cut each potato in half lengthwise and scoop out the flesh, leaving a thin layer of sweet potato attached to the skin.

5. In a bowl, mash the scooped•out sweet potato flesh. Add the shredded barbecue chicken and mix well.

6. Spoon the chicken and sweet potato mixture back into the potato skins. Top each stuffed potato with a sprinkle of shredded cheddar cheese.

7. Return the stuffed potatoes to the oven and bake for an additional 10•15 minutes, or until the cheese is melted and bubbly.

8. Garnish the stuffed sweet potatoes with chopped fresh cilantro, if desired.

9. Serve the BBQ Chicken Stuffed Sweet Potatoes immediately and enjoy!

This dish is a great source of complex carbohydrates, lean protein, and healthy fats, making it a nutritious and satisfying meal for both men and women. The combination of sweet potatoes, barbecue chicken, and melted cheese creates a delicious and flavorful dish.

9. Teriyaki Salmon with Broccoli

Ingredient:

• 4 (6 oz) salmon fillets
• 1/4 cup low•sodium teriyaki sauce
• 1 tbsp honey
• 1 tsp sesame oil
• 1 tsp grated fresh ginger
• 2 cloves garlic, minced
• 1 lb broccoli florets
• 1 tbsp olive oil
• Salt and pepper to taste
• Sesame seeds for garnish (optional)

Instructions:

1. Preheat your oven to 400°F (200°C). Line a baking sheet with parchment paper or a silicone baking mat.

2. In a small bowl, whisk together the teriyaki sauce, honey, sesame oil, grated ginger, and minced garlic.

3. Place the salmon fillets on the prepared baking sheet and brush the top of each fillet with the teriyaki sauce mixture, reserving any remaining sauce.

4. Roast the salmon in the preheated oven for 12•15 minutes, or until it flakes easily with a fork.

5. While the salmon is cooking, steam the broccoli florets until they are tender•crisp, about 5•7 minutes.

6. Drain the broccoli and transfer it to a large bowl. Drizzle the broccoli with the remaining teriyaki sauce mixture and the olive oil, and toss to coat.

7. Serve the Teriyaki Salmon fillets immediately, with the broccoli on the side. Garnish with sesame seeds, if desired.

This Teriyaki Salmon with Broccoli dish is a great source of lean protein, healthy fats, and fiber•rich vegetables. The sweet and savory teriyaki sauce complements the rich salmon perfectly, making it a delicious and satisfying meal for both men and women.

10. Protein·Packed Breakfast Burritos

Ingredient:

- 8 eggs, scrambled
- 1/2 lb lean ground turkey or turkey sausage, cooked and crumbled
- 1 cup black beans, rinsed and drained
- 1/2 cup shredded cheddar cheese
- 1/4 cup diced onion
- 1 tbsp olive oil
- Salt and pepper to taste
- 8 whole wheat tortillas

Instructions:

1. In a large skillet, cook the ground turkey or turkey sausage over medium heat until browned and cooked through, about 5·7 minutes. Drain any excess fat and set the cooked meat aside.

2. In the same skillet, heat the olive oil over medium heat. Add the diced onion and sauté for 2·3 minutes, until translucent.

3. Add the scrambled eggs to the skillet with the onions. Season with salt and pepper and cook, stirring occasionally, until the eggs are fully cooked, about 3·5 minutes.

4. Remove the skillet from the heat and stir in the cooked ground turkey or sausage and the black beans.

5. Warm the whole wheat tortillas according to the package instructions.

6. Spoon the egg, meat, and bean mixture onto the center of each tortilla. Top with a sprinkle of shredded cheddar cheese.

7. Fold the bottom of the tortilla up, then fold in the sides and roll up tightly to create a burrito.

8. Wrap the burritos individually in foil or parchment paper, and store them in the refrigerator or freezer for easy grab·and·go breakfasts.

These Protein·Packed Breakfast Burritos are a great option for both men and women who are looking for a nutritious and satisfying start to their day. The combination of eggs, lean protein, and fiber·rich beans and vegetables provides a balanced and filling meal.

11. Thai Peanut Chicken

Ingredient:

- 1/4 cup low•sodium soy sauce
- 2 tbsp rice vinegar
- 1 tbsp honey
- 1 tsp red pepper flakes (or more to taste)
- 1/4 cup chopped fresh cilantro
- 2 green onions, sliced
- Cooked brown rice or quinoa, for serving
- 1 lb boneless, skinless chicken breasts, cut into 1•inch pieces
- 2 tbsp olive oil
- 1 red bell pepper, sliced
- 1 cup snow peas or snap peas
- 2 cloves garlic, minced
- 1 tbsp grated fresh ginger
- 1/2 cup creamy peanut butter

Instructions:

1. In a large skillet or wok, heat the olive oil over medium•high heat.

2. Add the chicken pieces and stir•fry for 3•4 minutes, until the chicken is lightly browned.

3. Add the sliced red bell pepper and snow peas or snap peas to the skillet. Stir•fry for an additional 2•3 minutes, until the vegetables are tender•crisp.

4. Stir in the minced garlic and grated ginger, and cook for 1 minute, until fragrant.

5. In a small bowl, whisk together the peanut butter, soy sauce, rice vinegar, honey, and red pepper flakes.

6. Pour the peanut sauce into the skillet with the chicken and vegetables. Stir to coat everything evenly and cook for 2•3 minutes, until the sauce thickens slightly.

7. Remove the skillet from the heat and stir in the chopped cilantro and sliced green onions.

8. Serve the Thai Peanut Chicken immediately, over a bed of cooked brown rice or quinoa.

This Thai Peanut Chicken dish is a delicious and nutritious meal that can be enjoyed by both men and women. The combination of lean protein, fresh vegetables, and a creamy peanut sauce creates a flavorful and satisfying dish.

12. Blackened Tilapia with Mango Salsa

Ingredient:

For the Blackened Tilapia:
• 4 tilapia fillets
• 2 tablespoons blackened seasoning (or make your own blend with paprika, garlic powder, onion powder, cayenne, and salt)
• 2 tablespoons olive oil

For the Mango Salsa:
• 1 ripe mango, diced
• 1/2 red onion, finely chopped
• 1 jalapeño, seeded and finely chopped
• 1/4 cup chopped fresh cilantro
• 2 tablespoons freshly squeezed lime juice
• 1/4 teaspoon salt

Instructions:

1. Make the mango salsa: In a medium bowl, combine the diced mango, red onion, jalapeño, cilantro, lime juice, and salt. Stir to mix well and set aside.

2. Pat the tilapia fillets dry with paper towels and season both sides evenly with the blackened seasoning.

3. Heat the olive oil in a large skillet over medium•high heat. When the oil is hot, add the seasoned tilapia fillets and cook for 3•4 minutes per side, until the fish is opaque and flakes easily with a fork.

4. Transfer the blackened tilapia to plates or a serving platter. Top each fillet with a generous spoonful of the fresh mango salsa.

5. Serve the blackened tilapia immediately, with any extra mango salsa on the side.

This dish is a great option for both men and women. The blackened seasoning adds a bold, spicy flavor to the tender tilapia, while the sweet and tangy mango salsa provides a refreshing contrast. It's a healthy, protein•packed meal that's also full of vibrant colors and flavors. Enjoy!

13. Lemon Herb Grilled Chicken

Ingredient:

- 4 boneless, skinless chicken breasts
- 2 tablespoons olive oil
- 2 tablespoons freshly squeezed lemon juice
- 2 teaspoons lemon zest
- 2 cloves garlic, minced
- 1 tablespoon chopped fresh parsley
- 1 tablespoon chopped fresh thyme
- 1 teaspoon dried oregano
- 1/2 teaspoon salt
- 1/4 teaspoon black pepper

Instructions:

1. In a shallow baking dish or resealable plastic bag, combine the olive oil, lemon juice, lemon zest, garlic, parsley, thyme, oregano, salt, and pepper. Add the chicken breasts and turn to coat them evenly in the marinade.

2. Cover the dish or seal the bag and refrigerate for at least 30 minutes, or up to 4 hours.

3. Preheat your grill to medium•high heat.

4. Remove the chicken from the marinade and discard any remaining marinade.

5. Grill the chicken for 5•7 minutes per side, or until the internal temperature reaches 165°F.

6. Transfer the grilled chicken to a clean cutting board and let it rest for 5 minutes before slicing or serving.

Serve the Lemon Herb Grilled Chicken with your choice of sides, such as roasted vegetables, a fresh salad, or grilled asparagus. The bright, zesty flavors of the lemon and herbs complement the juicy, grilled chicken perfectly.

This recipe is a great option for both men and women, as it is a healthy, protein•rich meal that is also full of flavor. The marinade helps to keep the chicken moist and tender, making it a delicious and satisfying dish.

14. Veggie·Packed Turkey Chili

Ingredient:

- 1 lb ground turkey
- 1 tbsp olive oil
- 1 onion, diced
- 3 cloves garlic, minced
- 1 red bell pepper, diced
- 1 tsp dried oregano
- 1/2 tsp smoked paprika
- Salt and pepper to taste
- Chopped fresh cilantro for garnish (optional)

- 1 zucchini, diced
- 1 (15 oz) can diced tomatoes
- 1 (15 oz) can tomato sauce
- 1 (15 oz) can black beans, rinsed and drained
- 1 (15 oz) can kidney beans, rinsed and drained
- 2 tbsp chili powder
- 1 tsp ground cumin

Instructions:

1. In a large pot or Dutch oven, heat the olive oil over medium·high heat. Add the ground turkey and cook, breaking it up with a wooden spoon, until it's no longer pink, about 5·7 minutes.

2. Add the diced onion and minced garlic to the pot. Cook for 2·3 minutes, until the onion is translucent.

3. Stir in the diced red bell pepper and zucchini. Cook for an additional 3·4 minutes, until the vegetables start to soften.

4. Pour in the diced tomatoes, tomato sauce, rinsed and drained black beans and kidney beans, chili powder, cumin, oregano, and smoked paprika. Season with salt and pepper to taste.

5. Bring the chili to a simmer, then reduce the heat to low and let it cook for 20·25 minutes, stirring occasionally, until the flavors have melded and the vegetables are tender.

6. Serve the Veggie·Packed Turkey Chili hot, garnished with chopped fresh cilantro if desired. Serve with whole grain crackers, cornbread, or a side salad for a complete meal.

This chili is a great source of lean protein, fiber, and a variety of vegetables, making it a nutritious and satisfying dish for both men and women. The combination of spices and the addition of zucchini and bell pepper give it a delicious and well·rounded flavor.

15. Sweet Potato & Black Bean Enchiladas

Ingredient:

• 2 medium sweet potatoes, peeled and diced
• 1 tbsp olive oil
• 1 onion, diced
• 2 cloves garlic, minced
• 1 (15 oz) can black beans, rinsed and drained
• 1 tsp ground cumin
• 1 tsp chili powder
• Salt and pepper to taste
• 8 whole wheat tortillas
• 1 (15 oz) can enchilada sauce
• 1 cup shredded cheddar or Monterey Jack cheese

Instructions:

1. Preheat your oven to 375°F (190°C). Grease a 9x13 inch baking dish.

2. In a large skillet, heat the olive oil over medium heat. Add the diced sweet potatoes and sauté for 5•7 minutes, until they start to soften.

3. Add the diced onion and minced garlic to the skillet. Cook for an additional 2•3 minutes, until the onion is translucent.

4. Stir in the rinsed and drained black beans, ground cumin, chili powder, and a pinch of salt and pepper. Cook for 2•3 minutes, until the flavors are combined.

5. Spread about 1/2 cup of the sweet potato and black bean mixture onto the center of each whole wheat tortilla. Roll up the tortillas tightly and place them seam•side down in the prepared baking dish.

6. Pour the enchilada sauce evenly over the top of the rolled enchiladas. Sprinkle the shredded cheese over the top.

7. Bake the enchiladas in the preheated oven for 20•25 minutes, or until the cheese is melted and bubbly.

8. Serve the Sweet Potato & Black Bean Enchiladas hot, garnished with chopped cilantro, diced avocado, or a dollop of plain Greek yogurt, if desired.

This vegetarian dish is packed with fiber, complex carbohydrates, and plant•based protein, making it a nutritious and satisfying meal for both men and women. The combination of sweet potatoes, black beans, and enchilada sauce creates a delicious and flavorful dish.

16. Chicken Fajita Bowls

Ingredient:

• 1 lb boneless, skinless chicken breasts, sliced into strips
• 2 tablespoons olive oil
• 1 tablespoon fajita seasoning
 (or taco seasoning)
• 1 red bell pepper, sliced
• 1 green bell pepper, sliced
• 1 onion, sliced
• 2 cups cooked brown rice
• 1 avocado, diced
• 1 cup shredded cheddar or
 Monterey Jack cheese
• Chopped cilantro, for garnish
• Lime wedges, for serving

Fajita Seasoning:
• 1 teaspoon chili powder
• 1 teaspoon cumin
• 1 teaspoon garlic powder
• 1/2 teaspoon onion powder
• 1/2 teaspoon paprika
• 1/4 teaspoon cayenne pepper
• 1/4 teaspoon dried oregano
• 1/2 teaspoon salt
• 1/4 teaspoon black pepper

Instructions:
1. In a small bowl, mix together all the fajita seasoning ingredients.

2. In a large skillet, heat the olive oil over medium•high heat. Add the chicken and sprinkle with the fajita seasoning. Cook for 5•7 minutes, stirring occasionally, until the chicken is cooked through.

3. Add the sliced bell peppers and onion to the skillet. Cook for 5•7 minutes, stirring occasionally, until the vegetables are tender•crisp.

4. Divide the cooked brown rice evenly among 4 bowls. Top each bowl with the chicken and vegetable mixture, avocado, shredded cheese, and chopped cilantro.

5. Serve with lime wedges on the side.

These Chicken Fajita Bowls are a healthy, flavorful, and satisfying meal. The combination of seasoned chicken, sautéed peppers and onions, rice, avocado, and cheese creates a delicious and balanced dish. It's perfect for both men and women looking for a nutritious and tasty meal.

17. Maple Dijon Glazed Pork Chops

Ingredient:

- 4 boneless pork chops, about 1•inch thick
- 2 tablespoons olive oil
- Salt and black pepper to taste

Maple Dijon Glaze:
- 2 tablespoons pure maple syrup
- 2 tablespoons Dijon mustard
- 1 tablespoon apple cider vinegar
- 1 garlic clove, minced
- 1/4 teaspoon dried thyme
- 1/4 teaspoon salt
- 1/8 teaspoon black pepper

Instructions:

1. Preheat oven to 400°F.

2. Season the pork chops all over with salt and pepper.

3. In a large oven•safe skillet or cast•iron pan, heat the olive oil over medium•high heat. Sear the pork chops for 2•3 minutes per side until nicely browned.

4. In a small bowl, whisk together all the ingredients for the Maple Dijon Glaze.

5. Transfer the seared pork chops to the oven and bake for 8•10 minutes.

6. Remove the pork chops from the oven and brush the Maple Dijon Glaze all over the tops and sides of the chops.

7. Return the pork chops to the oven and bake for an additional 5•7 minutes, or until the pork chops reach an internal temperature of 145°F.

8. Let the pork chops rest for 5 minutes before serving. Spoon any remaining glaze from the pan over the top.

Serve the Maple Dijon Glazed Pork Chops with your choice of sides, such as roasted vegetables, mashed potatoes, or a fresh salad. The sweet and tangy glaze complements the savory pork perfectly, making this an appealing and satisfying meal for both men and women.

18. Baked Cod with Asparagus

Ingredient:

- 1 lb cod fillets, cut into 4 portions
- 1 lb asparagus, trimmed
- 2 tablespoons olive oil, divided
- 1 teaspoon lemon zest
- 2 tablespoons freshly squeezed lemon juice
- 2 cloves garlic, minced
- 1/4 teaspoon salt
- 1/4 teaspoon black pepper
- 2 tablespoons grated Parmesan cheese (optional)
- Lemon wedges for serving

Instructions:

1. Preheat your oven to 400°F. Line a large baking sheet with parchment paper or foil.

2. In a large bowl, toss the asparagus with 1 tablespoon of the olive oil, salt, and pepper. Spread the asparagus in a single layer on one side of the prepared baking sheet.

3. In a small bowl, mix together the remaining 1 tablespoon of olive oil, lemon zest, lemon juice, and garlic.

4. Place the cod fillets on the other side of the baking sheet. Brush or spoon the lemon•garlic mixture over the top of the cod.

5. Bake for 12•15 minutes, or until the cod is opaque and flakes easily with a fork and the asparagus is tender•crisp.

6. Optional: Sprinkle the Parmesan cheese over the cod during the last 2•3 minutes of baking.

7. Serve the baked cod immediately, with the roasted asparagus and lemon wedges on the side.

This Baked Cod with Asparagus is a simple, healthy, and delicious meal that is suitable for both men and women. The cod is flaky and tender, while the asparagus provides a nice crunch and freshness. The lemon•garlic topping adds bright, zesty flavor to the dish. It's a well•balanced meal that's easy to prepare and full of nutrients.

19. Lentil & Veggie Stew

Ingredient:

• 1 cup dry brown or green lentils, rinsed
• 4 cups vegetable broth
• 1 tablespoon olive oil
• 1 onion, diced
• 3 cloves garlic, minced
• 2 carrots, peeled and diced
• 2 celery stalks, diced
• 1 red bell pepper, diced
• 1 (14.5 oz) can diced tomatoes
• 2 teaspoons dried thyme
• 1 teaspoon dried oregano
• 1/2 teaspoon smoked paprika
• Salt and black pepper to taste
• Chopped parsley for garnish (optional)

Instructions:

1. In a large pot, bring the vegetable broth to a boil over high heat. Add the lentils, reduce heat to medium•low, and simmer for 15•20 minutes until lentils are tender. Drain and set aside.

2. In the same pot, heat the olive oil over medium heat. Add the onion and sauté for 3•4 minutes until translucent.

3. Add the garlic, carrots, celery, and bell pepper. Sauté for 5•7 minutes, stirring occasionally, until vegetables are tender.

4. Stir in the cooked lentils, diced tomatoes, thyme, oregano, and smoked paprika. Season with salt and pepper to taste.

5. Bring the stew to a simmer and let cook for 10•15 minutes, allowing the flavors to meld. Serve hot, garnished with chopped parsley if desired. Enjoy!

This hearty, veggie•packed stew is a nutritious and satisfying meal for both men and women. The lentils provide plant•based protein, while the vegetables offer fiber, vitamins, and minerals. It's a comforting and flavorful dish that can be enjoyed year•round.

20. Almond·Crusted Chicken Tenders

Ingredient:

- 1 lb boneless, skinless chicken tenders
- 1 cup sliced almonds
- 1/2 cup whole wheat breadcrumbs
- 1 teaspoon garlic powder
- 1 teaspoon paprika
- 1/2 teaspoon salt
- 1/4 teaspoon black pepper
- 2 eggs, beaten
- Olive oil cooking spray

Dipping Sauce (optional):
- 1/2 cup plain Greek yogurt
- 2 tablespoons Dijon mustard
- 1 tablespoon honey
- 1 tablespoon chopped fresh parsley

Instructions:

1. Preheat your oven to 400°F. Line a baking sheet with parchment paper or a silicone baking mat.

2. In a food processor, pulse the sliced almonds until they are finely chopped, but not a powder. Transfer the chopped almonds to a shallow bowl and mix in the breadcrumbs, garlic powder, paprika, salt, and pepper.

3. Dip the chicken tenders into the beaten eggs, allowing any excess to drip off. Then dredge the chicken in the almond·breadcrumb mixture, pressing gently to help it adhere.

4. Arrange the coated chicken tenders on the prepared baking sheet. Lightly spray the tops of the chicken with olive oil cooking spray.

5. Bake for 15·18 minutes, flipping halfway through, until the chicken is cooked through and the coating is golden brown.

6. While the chicken is baking, make the optional dipping sauce by whisking together the Greek yogurt, Dijon mustard, honey, and chopped parsley.

7. Serve the almond·crusted chicken tenders warm, with the dipping sauce on the side.

These Almond·Crusted Chicken Tenders are a delicious and healthy option that both men and women can enjoy. The almond coating provides a satisfying crunch, while the chicken remains juicy and tender. Serve it with a fresh salad or roasted vegetables for a complete and balanced meal.

21. Pesto Zucchini Noodles with Shrimp

Ingredient:

- 3 medium zucchini, spiralized or julienned into noodles
- 1 lb shrimp, peeled and deveined
- 2 tablespoons olive oil, divided
- 3 cloves garlic, minced
- 1/4 cup basil pesto (store•bought or homemade)
- 1/4 cup grated Parmesan cheese
- Salt and black pepper to taste
- Lemon wedges for serving (optional)

Instructions:

1. In a large skillet, heat 1 tablespoon of the olive oil over medium•high heat. Add the shrimp and garlic, and sauté for 2•3 minutes until the shrimp are opaque and cooked through. Transfer the shrimp and garlic to a plate and set aside.

2. In the same skillet, heat the remaining 1 tablespoon of olive oil over medium•high heat. Add the spiralized or julienned zucchini noodles and sauté for 2•3 minutes, just until the noodles are tender•crisp.

3. Remove the skillet from the heat and stir in the basil pesto and Parmesan cheese. Toss the zucchini noodles to coat them evenly.

4. Add the cooked shrimp and garlic back to the skillet and gently toss everything together.

5. Season the pesto zucchini noodles and shrimp with salt and black pepper to taste.

6. Serve the dish immediately, with lemon wedges on the side if desired.

This Pesto Zucchini Noodles with Shrimp recipe is a healthy, low•carb, and flavorful meal that can be enjoyed by both men and women. The zucchini noodles provide a nutritious alternative to traditional pasta, while the shrimp adds a lean protein source. The basil pesto and Parmesan cheese create a delicious, creamy sauce that ties the dish together. It's a quick and easy meal that's perfect for a weeknight dinner or a light, satisfying lunch.

22. Quinoa Stuffed Bell Peppers

Ingredient:

• 4 bell peppers (any color), halved lengthwise and seeds removed
• 1 cup cooked quinoa
• 1 (15 oz) can black beans, drained and rinsed
• 1 cup diced tomatoes
• 1/2 cup crumbled feta cheese
• 1/4 cup chopped fresh parsley
• 2 cloves garlic, minced
• 1 teaspoon ground cumin
• 1/2 teaspoon chili powder
• Salt and black pepper to taste
• Shredded cheddar cheese for topping (optional)

Instructions:

1. Preheat your oven to 375°F. Arrange the bell pepper halves in a baking dish or on a rimmed baking sheet.

2. In a large bowl, combine the cooked quinoa, black beans, diced tomatoes, feta cheese, parsley, garlic, cumin, chili powder, salt, and black pepper. Stir until well mixed.

3. Spoon the quinoa mixture evenly into the hollowed•out bell pepper halves.

4. If desired, top the stuffed peppers with shredded cheddar cheese.

5. Bake the stuffed peppers for 25•30 minutes, or until the peppers are tender and the filling is hot.

6. Serve the quinoa stuffed bell peppers warm.

These Quinoa Stuffed Bell Peppers are a nutritious and flavorful meal that can be enjoyed by both men and women. The combination of protein•rich quinoa, fiber•filled black beans, and fresh vegetables makes it a well•balanced dish. The feta cheese and spices add a delicious savory element.

This recipe is versatile, as you can use any color of bell pepper and adjust the fillings to your taste. It's a great option for a healthy, meatless main course or a satisfying side dish. Enjoy!

23. Spicy Chickpea & Spinach Curry

Ingredient:

- 2 tablespoons olive oil
- 1 onion, diced
- 3 cloves garlic, minced
- 1 tablespoon grated fresh ginger
- 1 tablespoon garam masala
- 1/4 cup chopped fresh cilantro
- Salt and black pepper to taste
- Cooked basmati rice, for serving

- 1 teaspoon ground cumin
- 1 teaspoon ground coriander
- 1/2 teaspoon cayenne pepper (or to taste)
- 1 (15 oz) can chickpeas, drained and rinsed
- 1 (14 oz) can diced tomatoes
- 1 cup vegetable broth
- 5 oz baby spinach

Instructions:

1. In a large skillet or Dutch oven, heat the olive oil over medium heat. Add the diced onion and sauté for 5•7 minutes until translucent.

2. Add the minced garlic and grated ginger to the pan. Cook for 1 minute, until fragrant.

3. Stir in the garam masala, cumin, coriander, and cayenne pepper. Cook for 1•2 minutes to toast the spices.

4. Add the drained and rinsed chickpeas, diced tomatoes, and vegetable broth. Bring the mixture to a simmer and let it cook for 10•15 minutes, allowing the flavors to meld.

5. Stir in the baby spinach and chopped cilantro. Cook for 2•3 minutes, until the spinach is wilted.

6. Season the curry with salt and black pepper to taste.

7. Serve the spicy chickpea and spinach curry over cooked basmati rice.

This Spicy Chickpea & Spinach Curry is a flavorful, vegetarian•friendly dish that can be enjoyed by both men and women. The combination of protein•rich chickpeas, nutrient•dense spinach, and aromatic spices creates a satisfying and wholesome meal. Adjust the amount of cayenne pepper to suit your desired level of heat. Enjoy!

24. Turkey & Spinach Stuffed Mushrooms

Ingredient:

- 12 oz cremini or button mushrooms, stems removed and finely chopped
- 1 lb ground turkey
- 2 cups fresh spinach, chopped
- 1/2 cup grated Parmesan cheese
- 2 cloves garlic, minced
- 1 teaspoon dried oregano
- 1/4 teaspoon red pepper flakes (optional)
- Salt and black pepper to taste

Instructions:

1. Preheat your oven to 375°F. Lightly grease a baking sheet or oven•safe dish.

2. Remove the stems from the mushrooms and finely chop them. Set the mushroom caps aside.

3. In a large skillet over medium heat, cook the ground turkey, breaking it up with a wooden spoon, until no longer pink, about 5•7 minutes.

4. Add the chopped mushroom stems, spinach, Parmesan, garlic, oregano, and red pepper flakes (if using) to the skillet. Cook for 2•3 minutes, stirring frequently, until the spinach is wilted.

5. Season the turkey and spinach mixture with salt and black pepper to taste.

6. Arrange the mushroom caps on the prepared baking sheet or dish. Spoon the turkey and spinach filling evenly into the mushroom caps.

7. Bake the stuffed mushrooms for 15•20 minutes, or until the mushrooms are tender and the filling is hot.

8. Serve the turkey and spinach stuffed mushrooms warm.

These Turkey & Spinach Stuffed Mushrooms make a delicious and healthy appetizer or snack that can be enjoyed by both men and women. The savory turkey and spinach filling is a great source of protein, while the mushrooms provide a low•carb, nutrient•dense base. The Parmesan cheese and herbs add wonderful flavor. They're easy to prepare and perfect for entertaining or as a quick, satisfying bite.

25. Cinnamon Apple Protein Pancakes

Ingredient:

- 1 cup rolled oats
- 1 scoop (about 30g) vanilla protein powder
- 1 teaspoon baking powder
- 1/2 teaspoon ground cinnamon
- 1/4 teaspoon salt
- 1 cup unsweetened almond milk
- 1 egg
- 1 tablespoon maple syrup
- 1 teaspoon vanilla extract
- 1 apple, peeled, cored and diced

Toppings:
- Additional maple syrup
- Chopped walnuts or pecans (optional)

Instructions:

1. In a blender, combine the rolled oats, protein powder, baking powder, cinnamon, and salt. Blend until the oats are finely ground into a flour•like consistency.

2. Add the almond milk, egg, maple syrup, and vanilla extract to the blender. Blend until the batter is smooth and well combined.

3. Fold the diced apple into the pancake batter.

4. Heat a large non•stick skillet or griddle over medium heat. Lightly grease the surface with cooking spray or a small amount of oil.

5. Scoop the batter onto the hot surface, using about 1/4 cup for each pancake. Cook for 2•3 minutes per side, or until golden brown.

6. Serve the cinnamon apple protein pancakes warm, drizzled with additional maple syrup and topped with chopped nuts, if desired.

These Cinnamon Apple Protein Pancakes are a nutritious and delicious breakfast option that can be enjoyed by both men and women. The oats and protein powder provide complex carbs and protein to help fuel your day, while the apples and cinnamon add natural sweetness and flavor. They're a great way to start your morning with a balanced and satisfying meal.

28. Teriyaki Turkey Meatballs

Ingredient:

- 1 lb ground turkey
- 1/2 cup panko breadcrumbs
- 1/4 cup finely chopped green onions
- 2 tablespoons low•sodium soy sauce
- 1 tablespoon sesame oil
- 1 teaspoon grated fresh ginger
- 1 clove garlic, minced
- 1/4 teaspoon salt
- 1/4 teaspoon black pepper

Teriyaki Sauce:

- 1/2 cup low•sodium soy sauce
- 1/4 cup brown sugar
- 2 tablespoons rice vinegar
- 1 tablespoon sesame oil
- 1 teaspoon cornstarch
- 1 clove garlic, minced
- 1/2 teaspoon ground ginger

Instructions:

1. Preheat your oven to 400°F. Line a baking sheet with parchment paper.

2. In a large bowl, combine the ground turkey, panko, green onions, soy sauce, sesame oil, ginger, garlic, salt, and pepper. Mix until just combined, being careful not to overmix.

3. Roll the turkey mixture into 1•inch meatballs and place them on the prepared baking sheet.

4. Bake the meatballs for 18•20 minutes, or until they are cooked through and no longer pink in the center.

5. While the meatballs are baking, make the teriyaki sauce. In a small saucepan, whisk together the soy sauce, brown sugar, rice vinegar, sesame oil, cornstarch, garlic, and ginger. Bring the mixture to a simmer and cook for 2•3 minutes, until thickened slightly.

6. Remove the meatballs from the oven and transfer them to a serving bowl. Pour the teriyaki sauce over the meatballs and gently toss to coat.

7. Serve the teriyaki turkey meatballs warm, garnished with additional green onions if desired. Enjoy!

These Teriyaki Turkey Meatballs are a delicious and healthy option that both men and women can enjoy. The lean ground turkey keeps the meatballs light, while the teriyaki sauce provides a flavorful, sweet•and•savory glaze. Serve them as an appetizer or as a main dish with steamed rice and vegetables.

29. Egg White & Veggie Muffins

Ingredient:

- 8 egg whites
- 1/2 cup diced bell pepper
- 1/2 cup diced onion
- 1/2 cup diced mushrooms
- 1/4 cup shredded spinach
- 2 tablespoons grated Parmesan cheese
- 1/4 teaspoon salt
- 1/8 teaspoon black pepper

Instructions:

1. Preheat your oven to 350°F. Grease a 12•cup muffin tin or line it with silicone or paper liners.

2. In a large bowl, whisk the egg whites until they are slightly frothy.

3. Add the diced bell pepper, onion, mushrooms, and shredded spinach to the egg whites. Stir to combine.

4. Divide the egg white and veggie mixture evenly among the prepared muffin cups, filling each one about 3/4 full.

5. Sprinkle the top of each muffin with a small amount of grated Parmesan cheese.

6. Bake the egg white and veggie muffins for 20•25 minutes, or until they are set and lightly golden on top.

7. Allow the muffins to cool in the tin for 5 minutes before removing them. Serve warm.

These Egg White & Veggie Muffins are a great healthy breakfast or snack option for both men and women. They are high in protein from the egg whites, and packed with nutrient•dense vegetables. The Parmesan cheese adds a nice savory flavor.

These muffins are easy to make and perfect for meal prep. You can store them in the refrigerator for up to 4 days or freeze them for longer•term storage. Reheat them in the microwave or oven when ready to enjoy.

The versatile veggie combination can be customized to your liking. Enjoy these egg white muffins as part of a balanced breakfast or as a satisfying snack throughout the day.

30. Grilled Lemon Herb Shrimp

Ingredient:

• 1 lb large shrimp, peeled and deveined
• 2 tablespoons olive oil
• 2 tablespoons freshly squeezed lemon juice
• 2 cloves garlic, minced
• 1 tablespoon chopped fresh parsley
• 1 tablespoon chopped fresh oregano
• 1/2 teaspoon salt
• 1/4 teaspoon black pepper
• Lemon wedges for serving

Instructions:

1. In a large bowl, combine the shrimp, olive oil, lemon juice, garlic, parsley, oregano, salt, and pepper. Toss to coat the shrimp evenly.

2. Preheat your grill or grill pan to medium•high heat.

3. Thread the marinated shrimp onto metal or wooden skewers, leaving a little space between each shrimp.

4. Grill the shrimp skewers for 2•3 minutes per side, or until the shrimp are opaque and cooked through.

5. Transfer the grilled lemon herb shrimp to a serving platter. Serve immediately with lemon wedges on the side.

This Grilled Lemon Herb Shrimp recipe is a great option for both men and women. The shrimp is packed with protein, while the bright, fresh flavors from the lemon, garlic, and herbs make it a light and flavorful dish.

Grilling the shrimp adds a nice smoky char and keeps the texture tender and juicy. Serve it as a main course with a side salad or roasted vegetables, or enjoy it as an appetizer or part of a larger seafood spread.

The simplicity of the recipe and the bold, crowd•pleasing flavors make this Grilled Lemon Herb Shrimp a versatile and appealing option for any occasion.

31. Sweet Potato & Turkey Shepherd's Pie

Ingredient:

- 1 lb ground turkey
- 1 onion, diced
- 2 cloves garlic, minced
- 1 cup diced carrots
- 1 cup frozen peas
- 1 cup frozen corn
- 2 tablespoons tomato paste
- 1 teaspoon dried thyme
- 1 teaspoon dried rosemary
- Salt and pepper to taste
- 3 medium sweet potatoes, peeled and cubed
- 2 tablespoons butter
- 1/4 cup milk
- 1/4 cup grated Parmesan cheese

Instructions:

1. Preheat your oven to 375°F (190°C).

2. In a large skillet over medium•high heat, cook the ground turkey, breaking it up with a wooden spoon, until browned, about 5•7 minutes. Drain any excess fat.

3. Add the diced onion and minced garlic to the skillet. Cook for 2•3 minutes, until the onion is translucent.

4. Stir in the diced carrots, frozen peas, frozen corn, tomato paste, thyme, rosemary, and season with salt and pepper. Cook for an additional 5 minutes.

5. Transfer the turkey and vegetable mixture to a 9x13 inch baking dish.

6. In a medium saucepan, cover the cubed sweet potatoes with water. Bring to a boil and cook until tender, about 15•20 minutes. Drain the sweet potatoes and mash them with the butter and milk until smooth.

7. Spread the mashed sweet potatoes evenly over the turkey and vegetable mixture in the baking dish. Sprinkle the Parmesan cheese on top.

8. Bake the shepherd's pie for 25•30 minutes, or until the sweet potato topping is lightly browned. Let the shepherd's pie cool for 5•10 minutes before serving.

32. Ginger Garlic Chicken Stir·Fry

Ingredient:

- 1 lb boneless, skinless chicken breasts, cut into 1·inch pieces
- 2 tablespoons vegetable or canola oil
- 3 cloves garlic, minced
- 1 tablespoon grated fresh ginger
- 1 red bell pepper, sliced
- 1 cup broccoli florets
- 1 cup sliced mushrooms
- 2 green onions, sliced
- 2 tablespoons low·sodium soy sauce
- 1 tablespoon rice vinegar
- 1 teaspoon sesame oil
- Salt and pepper to taste
- Cooked rice or noodles, for serving

Instructions:

1. Heat the vegetable oil in a large skillet or wok over high heat.

2. Add the chicken and cook, stirring occasionally, until lightly browned, about 3·4 minutes. Transfer the chicken to a plate.

3. Reduce the heat to medium and add the garlic and ginger to the skillet. Cook for 1 minute, stirring constantly, until fragrant.

4. Add the bell pepper, broccoli, and mushrooms to the skillet. Cook for 3·4 minutes, stirring frequently, until the vegetables are tender·crisp.

5. Return the chicken to the skillet and add the soy sauce, rice vinegar, and sesame oil. Toss everything together and cook for an additional 2·3 minutes, until the chicken is cooked through.

6. Remove from heat and stir in the sliced green onions. Season with salt and pepper to taste.

7. Serve the ginger garlic chicken stir·fry immediately over cooked rice or noodles.

Enjoy this flavorful and healthy stir·fry dish!

33. Spaghetti Squash Primavera

Ingredient:

- 1 medium spaghetti squash, halved lengthwise and seeds removed
- 2 tablespoons olive oil
- 1 cup diced zucchini
- 1 cup diced bell pepper (any color)
- 1 cup diced mushrooms
- 1/2 cup diced onion
- 3 cloves garlic, minced
- 1 cup cherry tomatoes, halved
- 1/4 cup grated Parmesan cheese
- 2 tablespoons chopped fresh basil
- Salt and pepper to taste

Instructions:

1. Preheat your oven to 400°F (200°C). Place the spaghetti squash halves cut•side down on a baking sheet. Bake for 30•40 minutes, or until the squash is tender and easily shreds with a fork.

2. While the squash is baking, heat the olive oil in a large skillet over medium heat. Add the zucchini, bell pepper, mushrooms, and onion. Sauté for 5•7 minutes, until the vegetables are tender.

3. Add the garlic to the skillet and cook for 1 minute, until fragrant.

4. Remove the spaghetti squash from the oven and let it cool slightly. Use a fork to shred the flesh into spaghetti•like strands.

5. Add the shredded spaghetti squash and the cherry tomatoes to the skillet with the sautéed vegetables. Toss everything together and cook for an additional 2•3 minutes, until the squash is heated through.

6. Remove the skillet from heat and stir in the Parmesan cheese and fresh basil. Season with salt and pepper to taste.

7. Serve the Spaghetti Squash Primavera warm, garnished with extra Parmesan and basil if desired.

Enjoy this healthy, veggie•packed twist on a classic pasta dish!

34. Greek Yogurt Chicken Salad

Ingredient:

- 2 cups cooked, shredded or diced chicken breast
- 1 cup plain Greek yogurt
- 1/4 cup diced celery
- 1/4 cup diced red onion
- 2 tablespoons chopped fresh dill
- 1 tablespoon Dijon mustard
- 1 tablespoon lemon juice
- Salt and pepper to taste

Instructions:

1. In a large bowl, combine the cooked, shredded or diced chicken, Greek yogurt, diced celery, diced red onion, chopped fresh dill, Dijon mustard, and lemon juice.

2. Stir everything together until well mixed.

3. Season with salt and pepper to taste.

4. Cover and refrigerate the chicken salad for at least 30 minutes to allow the flavors to meld.

5. Serve the Greek Yogurt Chicken Salad on a bed of greens, in a sandwich, or with crackers or sliced vegetables.

Tips:
- Use rotisserie chicken or leftover cooked chicken to save time.
- For a creamier texture, use full•fat Greek yogurt.
- Add grapes, diced apples, or toasted nuts for extra crunch and flavor.
- Adjust the amount of lemon juice and Dijon mustard to your taste preferences.

This Greek Yogurt Chicken Salad is a healthier, protein•packed alternative to traditional mayonnaise•based chicken salads. The Greek yogurt provides a creamy, tangy base, while the fresh dill, celery, and onion add flavor and crunch.

Enjoy this versatile chicken salad as a quick and nutritious lunch or snack!

35. Almond Butter Protein Smoothie

Ingredient:

• 1 cup unsweetened almond milk
• 1/2 cup plain Greek yogurt
• 2 tablespoons almond butter
• 1 scoop vanilla protein powder
• 1 frozen banana
• 1 tablespoon honey (optional)
• 1/2 teaspoon ground cinnamon

Instructions:

1. Add all the ingredients to a high•powered blender.

2. Blend on high speed until the mixture is smooth and creamy, about 1•2 minutes.

3. Taste and adjust sweetness by adding more honey if desired.

4. Pour the smoothie into a glass and enjoy immediately.

Tips:
• Use a ripe, frozen banana for a thicker, creamier texture.
• Adjust the amount of almond milk to reach your desired consistency.
• For a thicker smoothie, use less almond milk. For a thinner smoothie, add more.
• You can also add a handful of spinach or kale for extra nutrients.
• Customize the flavor by using different protein powder varieties, such as chocolate or peanut butter.

This Almond Butter Protein Smoothie is a great way to start your day with a nutritious and filling breakfast. The combination of almond butter, protein powder, and Greek yogurt provides a good source of protein, healthy fats, and fiber to keep you energized throughout the morning.

36. Baked Parmesan Zucchini Fries

Ingredient:

- 2 medium zucchini, cut into 1/4•inch thick fry•shaped pieces
- 1/2 cup grated Parmesan cheese
- 1/4 cup all•purpose flour
- 1 teaspoon garlic powder
- 1/2 teaspoon dried oregano
- 1/4 teaspoon salt
- 1/4 teaspoon black pepper
- 1 large egg, beaten

Instructions:

1. Preheat your oven to 400°F (200°C). Line a baking sheet with parchment paper or a silicone baking mat.

2. In a shallow bowl, combine the grated Parmesan cheese, flour, garlic powder, dried oregano, salt, and black pepper. Mix well.

3. In a separate shallow bowl, beat the egg.

4. Dip the zucchini fry pieces into the beaten egg, allowing any excess to drip off.

5. Transfer the egg•coated zucchini fries to the Parmesan cheese mixture and toss to coat them evenly.

6. Arrange the coated zucchini fries in a single layer on the prepared baking sheet.

7. Bake for 18•22 minutes, flipping the fries halfway through, until they are golden brown and crispy.

8. Remove the baked Parmesan zucchini fries from the oven and serve immediately, while hot.

Tips:
- For extra crispiness, you can spritz the fries with a little olive oil or cooking spray before baking.
- Adjust the baking time as needed, depending on the thickness of your zucchini fries.
- Serve the Parmesan zucchini fries with your favorite dipping sauce, such as marinara, ranch, or garlic aioli.

37. Buffalo Cauliflower Bites

Ingredient:

- 1 head of cauliflower, cut into bite•sized florets
- 1/2 cup all•purpose flour
- 1/2 cup unsweetened almond milk (or regular milk)
- 1 teaspoon garlic powder
- 1/2 teaspoon onion powder
- 1/4 teaspoon cayenne pepper
- 1/4 teaspoon salt
- 1/2 cup buffalo sauce (such as Frank's RedHot)
- 2 tablespoons melted butter or olive oil

Instructions:

1. Preheat your oven to 400°F (200°C). Line a baking sheet with parchment paper.

2. In a large bowl, whisk together the flour, almond milk, garlic powder, onion powder, cayenne pepper, and salt until a smooth batter forms.

3. Add the cauliflower florets to the batter and toss to coat them evenly.

4. Arrange the battered cauliflower florets in a single layer on the prepared baking sheet.

5. Bake for 20•25 minutes, flipping the florets halfway through, until the batter is crispy and the cauliflower is tender.

6. In a separate bowl, whisk together the buffalo sauce and melted butter or olive oil.

7. Remove the baked cauliflower florets from the oven and transfer them to the buffalo sauce mixture. Toss to coat the florets evenly.

8. Return the coated cauliflower bites to the baking sheet and bake for an additional 5•10 minutes, until the sauce has thickened and the bites are crispy.

9. Serve the Buffalo Cauliflower Bites warm, with your favorite dipping sauce (such as ranch or blue cheese dressing) on the side.

Enjoy these spicy, flavorful, and healthier alternative to traditional buffalo wings!

38. Citrus Herb Roasted Salmon

Ingredient:

- 1 lb salmon fillets, skin•on or skinless
- 2 tablespoons olive oil
- 2 tablespoons freshly squeezed orange juice
- 1 tablespoon freshly squeezed lemon juice
- 2 cloves garlic, minced
- 1 tablespoon chopped fresh parsley
- 1 tablespoon chopped fresh dill
- 1 teaspoon grated orange zest
- 1/2 teaspoon salt
- 1/4 teaspoon black pepper

Instructions:

1. Preheat your oven to 400°F. Line a baking sheet with parchment paper or foil.

2. Place the salmon fillets on the prepared baking sheet, skin•side down if using skin•on salmon.

3. In a small bowl, whisk together the olive oil, orange juice, lemon juice, garlic, parsley, dill, orange zest, salt, and black pepper.

4. Drizzle the citrus herb mixture evenly over the top of the salmon fillets, making sure to coat them completely.

5. Roast the salmon in the preheated oven for 12•15 minutes, or until the fish flakes easily with a fork and is cooked through.

6. Optionally, you can broil the salmon for the last 2•3 minutes to get a nice caramelized top. Serve the Citrus Herb Roasted Salmon immediately, garnished with additional fresh herbs if desired.

This Citrus Herb Roasted Salmon is a delicious and healthy meal that can be enjoyed by both men and women. The bright, zesty flavors from the orange, lemon, and herbs complement the rich, flaky salmon perfectly.

Salmon is an excellent source of omega•3 fatty acids, protein, and other essential nutrients. This recipe is easy to prepare and makes for a quick, weeknight•friendly dinner. Serve it with roasted vegetables, a fresh salad, or your favorite side dish for a complete and balanced meal.

39. Chickpea & Avocado Salad

Ingredient:

- 1 (15 oz) can chickpeas, drained and rinsed
- 1 ripe avocado, diced
- 1/2 cup diced cucumber
- 1/4 cup diced red onion
- 2 tablespoons chopped fresh cilantro
- 2 tablespoons fresh lemon juice
- 1 tablespoon olive oil
- 1/4 teaspoon ground cumin
- Salt and pepper to taste

Instructions:

1. In a large bowl, gently combine the drained and rinsed chickpeas, diced avocado, diced cucumber, diced red onion, and chopped fresh cilantro.

2. In a small bowl, whisk together the lemon juice, olive oil, and ground cumin.

3. Pour the lemon•olive oil dressing over the chickpea and avocado mixture and gently toss to coat.

4. Season the salad with salt and pepper to taste.

5. Serve the Chickpea & Avocado Salad immediately or refrigerate until ready to serve.

Tips:
- For a creamier texture, you can mash half of the avocado before adding it to the salad.
- Add diced tomatoes or bell peppers for extra color and flavor.
- Swap the cilantro for parsley or basil if you prefer.
- Serve the salad on a bed of greens or with whole•grain crackers or pita bread.
- This salad can be made ahead of time and stored in the refrigerator for up to 3 days.

This Chickpea & Avocado Salad is a delicious, protein•packed, and nutrient•dense dish that makes a great lunch or light dinner. The combination of creamy avocado, protein•rich chickpeas, and fresh vegetables creates a satisfying and flavorful salad.

40. BBQ Chicken & Veggie Skewers

Ingredient:

- 1 lb boneless, skinless chicken breasts, cut into 1•inch cubes
- 1 red bell pepper, cut into 1•inch pieces
- 1 yellow bell pepper, cut into 1•inch pieces
- 1 red onion, cut into 1•inch pieces
- 8 oz mushrooms, halved
- 1/2 cup barbecue sauce (your favorite brand)
- 2 tablespoons olive oil
- Salt and pepper to taste
- Wooden or metal skewers

Instructions:

1. Preheat your grill or grill pan to medium•high heat.

2. In a large bowl, combine the cubed chicken, bell pepper pieces, onion pieces, and mushrooms. Drizzle with the olive oil and toss to coat.

3. Season the chicken and vegetables with salt and pepper to taste.

4. Thread the chicken and vegetables onto the skewers, alternating the ingredients.

5. Brush the skewered chicken and vegetables with the barbecue sauce, reserving some sauce for serving.

6. Grill the skewers for 12•15 minutes, turning occasionally, until the chicken is cooked through and the vegetables are tender.

7. Serve the BBQ Chicken & Veggie Skewers immediately, with the reserved barbecue sauce on the side for dipping.

Tips:
- Soak wooden skewers in water for 30 minutes before using to prevent them from burning.
- You can use a variety of vegetables, such as zucchini, cherry tomatoes, or pineapple chunks.
- Adjust the cooking time as needed, depending on the thickness of your chicken and vegetable pieces.
- For extra flavor, you can marinate the chicken in the barbecue sauce for 30 minutes to an hour before assembling the skewers.

41. Lemon Garlic Quinoa

Ingredient:

- 1 cup uncooked quinoa, rinsed
- 2 cups low•sodium vegetable or chicken broth
- 2 cloves garlic, minced
- 2 tablespoons fresh lemon juice
- 1 teaspoon grated lemon zest
- 2 tablespoons chopped fresh parsley
- Salt and pepper to taste

Instructions:

1. In a medium saucepan, combine the rinsed quinoa and broth. Bring the mixture to a boil over high heat.

2. Once boiling, reduce the heat to low, cover the saucepan with a lid, and simmer for 15•20 minutes, or until the quinoa is tender and the liquid is absorbed.

3. Remove the saucepan from the heat and fluff the quinoa with a fork.

4. Stir in the minced garlic, lemon juice, lemon zest, and chopped parsley. Season with salt and pepper to taste.

5. Serve the Lemon Garlic Quinoa warm or at room temperature.

Tips:
- Use freshly squeezed lemon juice for the best flavor.
- Adjust the amount of lemon juice and zest to your personal taste preferences.
- For extra flavor, you can sauté the garlic in a bit of olive oil before adding it to the quinoa.
- Garnish with additional chopped parsley or lemon wedges, if desired.

This Lemon Garlic Quinoa makes a great side dish or can be served as a light main course. The bright, citrusy flavors paired with the nutty quinoa and aromatic garlic create a delicious and nutritious meal.

Enjoy this flavorful and versatile quinoa dish!

42. Spicy Black Bean Burgers

Ingredient:

- 1 (15 oz) can black beans, drained and rinsed
- 1/2 cup cooked quinoa
- 1/2 cup breadcrumbs
- 1 egg, lightly beaten
- 2 tablespoons diced onion
- 2 cloves garlic, minced
- 1 jalapeño, seeded and minced
- 1 teaspoon chili powder
- 1/2 teaspoon cumin
- 1/4 teaspoon smoked paprika
- Salt and pepper to taste
- Olive oil or cooking spray for cooking

Instructions:

1. In a large bowl, mash the black beans with a fork or potato masher, leaving some texture.

2. Add the cooked quinoa, breadcrumbs, beaten egg, diced onion, minced garlic, minced jalapeño, chili powder, cumin, smoked paprika, and season with salt and pepper. Mix well until the ingredients are fully combined.

3. Divide the black bean mixture into 4•6 equal portions and shape them into patties, about 1/2 inch thick.

4. Heat a large skillet over medium heat and lightly coat with olive oil or cooking spray.

5. Cook the black bean burgers for 4•5 minutes per side, or until they are heated through and lightly browned.

6. Serve the Spicy Black Bean Burgers on whole•grain buns or lettuce wraps, with your favorite toppings such as avocado, tomato, onion, and a dollop of Greek yogurt or low•fat mayonnaise.

These Spicy Black Bean Burgers are a delicious and nutritious option for both men and women. They are packed with plant•based protein, fiber, and a kick of spice, making them a satisfying and healthy meal choice.

43. Veggie·Packed Egg Muffins

Ingredient:

- 12 large eggs
- 1/2 cup diced bell pepper (any color)
- 1/2 cup diced onion
- 1 cup chopped spinach or kale
- 1/4 cup shredded cheddar cheese (optional)
- Salt and pepper to taste

Instructions:

1. Preheat your oven to 350°F (175°C). Grease a 12·cup muffin tin or line it with paper liners.

2. In a large bowl, whisk the eggs together. Add the diced bell pepper, onion, and chopped spinach/kale. Season with salt and pepper.

3. Divide the egg mixture evenly among the prepared muffin cups, filling each about 3/4 full.

4. If using, sprinkle the shredded cheddar cheese on top of the egg mixture in each cup.

5. Bake for 20·25 minutes, or until the eggs are set and the tops are lightly golden.

6. Allow the egg muffins to cool in the tin for 5 minutes before removing them.

7. Serve warm or at room temperature. These egg muffins can be stored in the refrigerator for up to 4 days or frozen for longer storage.

Enjoy these nutrient·dense, veggie·packed egg muffins as a quick and easy breakfast or snack for both men and women!

44. Thai Basil Beef

Ingredient:

- 1 lb ground beef or ground turkey
- 2 tablespoons vegetable oil
- 3 cloves garlic, minced
- 1 tablespoon grated ginger
- 1 red bell pepper, sliced
- 1 cup sliced mushrooms
- 1/4 cup low•sodium soy sauce
- 2 tablespoons fish sauce
- 1 tablespoon brown sugar
- 1 teaspoon Sriracha or other hot sauce (optional)
- 1 cup fresh Thai basil leaves, chopped
- Cooked rice, for serving

Instructions:

1. In a large skillet or wok, heat the vegetable oil over medium•high heat.

2. Add the ground beef or turkey and cook, breaking it up with a wooden spoon, until browned and cooked through, about 5•7 minutes. Drain any excess fat.

3. Add the minced garlic and grated ginger to the skillet and cook for 1 minute, until fragrant.

4. Stir in the sliced red bell pepper and mushrooms. Cook for 2•3 minutes, until the vegetables are tender•crisp.

5. In a small bowl, whisk together the soy sauce, fish sauce, brown sugar, and Sriracha (if using).

6. Pour the sauce mixture into the skillet and stir to combine with the beef and vegetables.

7. Reduce the heat to low and let the sauce simmer for 2•3 minutes, until slightly thickened.

8. Remove the skillet from heat and stir in the chopped fresh Thai basil leaves. Serve the Thai Basil Beef immediately, over steamed rice.

45. Balsamic Glazed Brussels Sprouts

Ingredient:

• 1 lb Brussels sprouts, trimmed and halved
• 2 tablespoons olive oil
• 1/4 cup balsamic vinegar
• 2 tablespoons honey
• 1 clove garlic, minced
• 1/4 teaspoon salt
• 1/4 teaspoon black pepper

Instructions:

1. Preheat your oven to 400°F (200°C). Line a baking sheet with parchment paper.

2. In a large bowl, toss the trimmed and halved Brussels sprouts with the olive oil, making sure they are evenly coated.

3. Spread the Brussels sprouts in a single layer on the prepared baking sheet.

4. Roast the Brussels sprouts for 15•20 minutes, or until they are starting to become tender and lightly browned.

5. In a small bowl, whisk together the balsamic vinegar, honey, minced garlic, salt, and black pepper.

6. Remove the Brussels sprouts from the oven and drizzle the balsamic glaze over them, tossing to coat evenly.

7. Return the Brussels sprouts to the oven and continue roasting for an additional 10•15 minutes, or until the sprouts are tender and the glaze has thickened. Serve the Balsamic Glazed Brussels Sprouts immediately, while hot.

Tips:
• For extra crispiness, you can broil the Brussels sprouts for the last 2•3 minutes of cooking.
• Add chopped walnuts or pecans for a crunchy texture.
• Sprinkle with grated Parmesan cheese or crumbled feta for extra flavor.
• Adjust the amount of balsamic vinegar or honey to your taste preferences.

These Balsamic Glazed Brussels Sprouts make a delicious and healthy side dish. The sweet and tangy balsamic glaze perfectly complements the roasted Brussels sprouts, creating a flavorful and caramelized vegetable dish.

46. Chicken & Veggie Fajita Bowl

Ingredient:

- 1 lb boneless, skinless chicken breasts, sliced into strips
- 1 red bell pepper, sliced
- 1 yellow bell pepper, sliced
- 1 onion, sliced
- 2 tablespoons olive oil
- 2 tablespoons fajita seasoning
- 1 cup cooked brown rice
- 1 avocado, diced
- 1/4 cup shredded cheddar cheese
- Chopped cilantro, for garnish
- Lime wedges, for serving

Fajita Seasoning:
- 1 teaspoon chili powder
- 1 teaspoon cumin
- 1/2 teaspoon garlic powder
- 1/2 teaspoon onion powder
- 1/4 teaspoon smoked paprika
- 1/4 teaspoon dried oregano
- 1/4 teaspoon salt
- 1/4 teaspoon black pepper

Instructions:

1. In a small bowl, mix together all the ingredients for the fajita seasoning.

2. In a large skillet or wok, heat the olive oil over medium•high heat.

3. Add the sliced chicken, bell peppers, and onion to the skillet. Sprinkle the fajita seasoning over the top and toss to coat the ingredients evenly.

4. Cook the fajita mixture, stirring occasionally, for 8•10 minutes, or until the chicken is cooked through and the vegetables are tender•crisp.

5. Divide the cooked brown rice among 4 bowls. Top each bowl with the chicken and vegetable fajita mixture, diced avocado, and shredded cheddar cheese.

6. Garnish the Chicken & Veggie Fajita Bowls with chopped cilantro and serve with lime wedges.

Tips:
- For a spicier version, add a diced jalapeño or a sprinkle of crushed red pepper flakes.
- Swap the brown rice for quinoa or cauliflower rice for a low•carb option.
- Add other toppings like diced tomatoes, sour cream, or salsa to customize the bowls.
- Meal prep the components separately and assemble the bowls when ready to serve.

47. Cranberry Almond Protein Bars

Ingredient:

- 1 cup rolled oats
- 1/2 cup almond flour
- 1/4 cup unflavored whey protein powder
- 1/4 cup chopped almonds
- 1/4 cup dried cranberries
- 1/4 cup honey
- 2 tablespoons peanut butter (or almond butter)
- 1 teaspoon vanilla extract
- 1/4 teaspoon salt

Instructions:

1. Preheat your oven to 325ºF (165ºC). Line an 8x8 inch baking pan with parchment paper, leaving some overhang on the sides for easy removal.

2. In a large bowl, combine the rolled oats, almond flour, whey protein powder, chopped almonds, and dried cranberries. Mix well.

3. In a separate bowl, whisk together the honey, peanut butter (or almond butter), vanilla extract, and salt until smooth.

4. Pour the honey•peanut butter mixture into the dry ingredients and stir until well combined.

5. Transfer the mixture to the prepared baking pan and press it down firmly and evenly with your hands or a spatula.

6. Bake for 18•22 minutes, or until the edges are lightly golden.

7. Remove the pan from the oven and let the bars cool completely in the pan.

8. Once cooled, lift the bars out of the pan using the parchment paper overhang. Cut into 12 equal•sized bars.

9. Store the Cranberry Almond Protein Bars in an airtight container at room temperature for up to 1 week, or in the refrigerator for up to 2 weeks.

These Cranberry Almond Protein Bars are a nutritious and satisfying snack or breakfast option for both men and women. The combination of protein, healthy fats, and complex carbohydrates makes them a great choice to fuel your day.

48. Spicy Sriracha Chicken

Ingredient:

- 1 lb boneless, skinless chicken breasts, cut into 1•inch pieces
- 2 tablespoons Sriracha sauce
- 2 tablespoons low•sodium soy sauce
- 1 tablespoon honey
- 2 cloves garlic, minced
- 1 teaspoon grated ginger
- 1 tablespoon vegetable or sesame oil
- 1/4 cup chopped green onions
- 2 tablespoons chopped cilantro (optional)
- Salt and pepper to taste

Instructions:

1. In a large bowl, combine the cubed chicken, Sriracha sauce, soy sauce, honey, minced garlic, and grated ginger. Toss to coat the chicken evenly.

2. Heat the vegetable or sesame oil in a large skillet or wok over medium•high heat.

3. Add the marinated chicken to the hot skillet and cook, stirring occasionally, until the chicken is cooked through and no longer pink, about 8•10 minutes.

4. Stir in the chopped green onions and cook for an additional 1•2 minutes.

5. Remove the skillet from heat and stir in the chopped cilantro, if using.

6. Season the Spicy Sriracha Chicken with salt and pepper to taste.

7. Serve the chicken immediately, over steamed rice, quinoa, or with your favorite sides.

Tips:
- Adjust the amount of Sriracha sauce to your desired level of spiciness.
- For a creamier texture, you can stir in a tablespoon of Greek yogurt or coconut milk at the end.
- Add diced bell peppers, mushrooms, or other vegetables to the skillet for a more complete meal.
- Garnish with additional green onions, cilantro, and a drizzle of Sriracha sauce.

49. Roasted Red Pepper Hummus

Ingredient:

- 1 (15 oz) can chickpeas, drained and rinsed
- 1/2 cup roasted red peppers, drained and patted dry
- 2 tablespoons tahini
- 2 tablespoons fresh lemon juice
- 2 cloves garlic, minced
- 1 teaspoon ground cumin
- 1/4 teaspoon smoked paprika
- 2•3 tablespoons water, as needed
- Salt and pepper to taste
- Chopped parsley or paprika for garnish (optional)

Instructions:

1. In a food processor or high•powered blender, combine the drained and rinsed chickpeas, roasted red peppers, tahini, lemon juice, minced garlic, cumin, and smoked paprika.

2. Pulse the mixture several times, then process or blend on high speed, scraping down the sides as needed, until the hummus is smooth and creamy.

3. If the hummus is too thick, add 1•2 tablespoons of water and blend again until you reach your desired consistency.

4. Taste the hummus and season with salt and pepper to your liking.

5. Transfer the Roasted Red Pepper Hummus to a serving bowl or container.

6. Garnish the hummus with chopped parsley or a light dusting of smoked paprika, if desired.

7. Serve the hummus with pita bread, fresh vegetables (such as carrots, cucumber, or bell pepper strips), or whole•grain crackers.

This Roasted Red Pepper Hummus is a delicious and nutritious dip or spread that can be enjoyed by both men and women. The combination of protein•rich chickpeas, healthy fats from the tahini, and the sweet and smoky flavors of the roasted red peppers make it a satisfying and versatile snack or appetizer.

50. Beef & Sweet Potato Hash

Ingredient:

- 1 lb ground beef
- 2 medium sweet potatoes, peeled and diced
- 1 onion, diced
- 2 cloves garlic, minced
- 1 red bell pepper, diced
- 1 teaspoon chili powder
- 1 teaspoon paprika
- 1/2 teaspoon cumin
- Salt and pepper to taste
- 2 tablespoons olive oil
- 2 eggs (optional)

Instructions:

1. In a large skillet or cast•iron pan, cook the ground beef over medium•high heat, breaking it up with a wooden spoon, until browned and cooked through, about 5•7 minutes. Drain any excess fat.

2. Add the diced sweet potatoes, onion, garlic, and red bell pepper to the skillet. Drizzle with the olive oil and season with the chili powder, paprika, cumin, salt, and pepper.

3. Cook the hash, stirring occasionally, until the sweet potatoes are tender and the vegetables are softened, about 15•20 minutes.

4. If desired, create two wells in the hash and crack the eggs into them. Cover the skillet and cook the eggs until the whites are set and the yolks are cooked to your desired doneness, about 5•7 minutes.

5. Remove the skillet from heat and serve the Beef & Sweet Potato Hash immediately, with the eggs on top if using.

Tips:
- For a spicier hash, add a diced jalapeño or crushed red pepper flakes.
- Swap the ground beef for ground turkey or Italian sausage for different flavor variations.
- Add chopped kale, spinach, or other greens for extra nutrition.
- Serve the hash with a side of avocado, salsa, or Greek yogurt.

51. Spinach & Feta Stuffed Chicken

Ingredient:

- 4 boneless, skinless chicken breasts
- 1 cup fresh spinach, chopped
- 1/2 cup crumbled feta cheese
- 2 cloves garlic, minced
- 1 tablespoon olive oil
- Salt and pepper to taste

Instructions:

1. Preheat your oven to 400°F (200°C). Grease a baking dish or line it with parchment paper.

2. Using a sharp knife, carefully slice each chicken breast horizontally to create a pocket, being careful not to cut all the way through.

3. In a small bowl, mix together the chopped spinach, crumbled feta cheese, and minced garlic.

4. Stuff the spinach•feta mixture evenly into the pockets of the chicken breasts.

5. Drizzle the stuffed chicken breasts with the olive oil and season with salt and pepper.

6. Place the stuffed chicken breasts in the prepared baking dish.

7. Bake the chicken for 25•30 minutes, or until the chicken is cooked through and the internal temperature reaches 165°F (75°C).

8. Remove the Spinach & Feta Stuffed Chicken from the oven and let it rest for 5 minutes before serving.

This Spinach & Feta Stuffed Chicken is a delicious and nutritious meal that can be enjoyed by both men and women. The combination of lean protein, healthy fats, and nutrient•dense spinach and feta makes it a well•balanced and satisfying dish.

Enjoy this Spinach & Feta Stuffed Chicken!

52. Ginger Lime Grilled Shrimp

Ingredient:

- 1 lb large shrimp, peeled and deveined
- 2 tablespoons olive oil
- 2 tablespoons freshly squeezed lime juice
- 1 tablespoon grated fresh ginger
- 2 cloves garlic, minced
- 1 teaspoon honey
- 1/4 teaspoon red pepper flakes (optional)
- Salt and pepper to taste
- Lime wedges for serving

Instructions:

1. In a large bowl, combine the shrimp, olive oil, lime juice, grated ginger, minced garlic, honey, and red pepper flakes (if using). Toss to coat the shrimp evenly.

2. Cover the bowl and refrigerate for 30 minutes to 1 hour, allowing the shrimp to marinate.

3. Preheat your grill or grill pan to medium·high heat.

4. Thread the marinated shrimp onto metal or wooden skewers, leaving a little space between each shrimp.

5. Grill the shrimp skewers for 2·3 minutes per side, or until the shrimp are opaque and cooked through.

6. Remove the grilled shrimp from the skewers and transfer to a serving platter.

7. Season the shrimp with salt and pepper to taste.

8. Serve the Ginger Lime Grilled Shrimp immediately, with lime wedges on the side.

This Ginger Lime Grilled Shrimp is a delicious and easy·to·make seafood dish that's perfect for summer grilling. The bright, tangy, and slightly spicy flavors of the marinade complement the sweet and juicy shrimp perfectly.

Enjoy this Ginger Lime Grilled Shrimp!

53. Roasted Butternut Squash Soup

Ingredient:

- 1 medium butternut squash, peeled, seeded, and cubed (about 4 cups)
- 1 onion, diced
- 2 cloves garlic, minced
- 2 tablespoons olive oil
- 4 cups low·sodium vegetable or chicken broth
- 1 teaspoon ground cumin
- 1/2 teaspoon ground cinnamon
- 1/4 teaspoon ground nutmeg
- Salt and pepper to taste
- Chopped parsley or pepitas for garnish (optional)

Instructions:

1. Preheat your oven to 400°F (200°C). Line a baking sheet with parchment paper.

2. In a large bowl, toss the cubed butternut squash, diced onion, and minced garlic with the olive oil. Season with a pinch of salt and pepper.

3. Spread the seasoned vegetables in a single layer on the prepared baking sheet.

4. Roast the vegetables for 25·30 minutes, or until the squash is tender and lightly caramelized, stirring halfway through.

5. In a large pot or Dutch oven, add the roasted vegetables and the vegetable or chicken broth. Bring the mixture to a boil over high heat.

6. Reduce the heat to medium·low and let the soup simmer for 10·15 minutes, or until the vegetables are very soft.

7. Using an immersion blender or a regular blender, puree the soup until smooth and creamy.

8. Return the pureed soup to the pot and stir in the ground cumin, cinnamon, and nutmeg. Season with additional salt and pepper to taste.

9. Serve the Roasted Butternut Squash Soup warm, garnished with chopped parsley or pepitas, if desired.

56. Cinnamon Sweet Potato Protein Bars

Ingredient:

• 1 cup mashed sweet potato (about 1 medium sweet potato)
• 1/2 cup oat flour
• 1/4 cup unflavored whey protein powder
• 1/4 cup unsweetened applesauce
• 2 tablespoons honey
• 1 teaspoon ground cinnamon
• 1/2 teaspoon baking powder
• 1/4 teaspoon salt

Instructions:

1. Preheat your oven to 350ºF (175ºC). Line an 8x8 inch baking pan with parchment paper, leaving some overhang on the sides for easy removal.

2. In a medium bowl, mash the sweet potato until smooth.

3. Add the oat flour, whey protein powder, unsweetened applesauce, honey, ground cinnamon, baking powder, and salt to the mashed sweet potato. Mix well until all the ingredients are fully incorporated.

4. Spread the sweet potato batter evenly into the prepared baking pan.

5. Bake the bars for 20•25 minutes, or until a toothpick inserted in the center comes out clean.

6. Allow the bars to cool completely in the pan before lifting them out using the parchment paper overhang.

7. Cut the cooled bars into 12 equal•sized pieces.

8. Store the Cinnamon Sweet Potato Protein Bars in an airtight container at room temperature for up to 5 days, or in the refrigerator for up to 1 week.

These Cinnamon Sweet Potato Protein Bars are a delicious and nutritious snack or breakfast option for both men and women. The combination of sweet potato, protein•rich whey powder, and warming cinnamon creates a satisfying and flavorful bar.

Enjoy these Cinnamon Sweet Potato Protein Bars!

57. Asian Chicken Lettuce Wraps

Ingredient:

- 1 lb ground chicken or turkey
- 2 tablespoons sesame oil
- 3 cloves garlic, minced
- 1 tablespoon grated fresh ginger
- 2 tablespoons low•sodium soy sauce
- 1 tablespoon rice vinegar
- 1 tablespoon honey
- 1 teaspoon Sriracha or other hot sauce (optional)
- 1 cup shredded carrots
- 1 cup thinly sliced mushrooms
- 1/2 cup chopped green onions
- 1/4 cup chopped fresh cilantro
- 12•16 large lettuce leaves (such as romaine, bibb, or butter lettuce)

Instructions:

1. In a large skillet or wok, cook the ground chicken or turkey over medium•high heat, breaking it up with a wooden spoon, until browned and cooked through, about 5•7 minutes. Drain any excess fat.

2. Add the sesame oil, minced garlic, and grated ginger to the skillet. Cook for 1 minute, stirring constantly, until fragrant.

3. Stir in the soy sauce, rice vinegar, honey, and Sriracha (if using). Bring the mixture to a simmer and cook for 2•3 minutes, until the sauce has thickened slightly.

4. Add the shredded carrots, sliced mushrooms, chopped green onions, and chopped cilantro to the skillet. Toss everything together and cook for an additional 2•3 minutes, until the vegetables are tender.

5. Remove the skillet from heat and let the filling cool slightly.

6. To serve, place a spoonful of the Asian chicken filling into the center of a lettuce leaf. Fold the lettuce leaf around the filling and enjoy.

These Asian Chicken Lettuce Wraps are a light, flavorful, and healthy meal option. The combination of savory, sweet, and spicy flavors in the filling, wrapped in crisp lettuce leaves, makes for a delicious and satisfying dish.

60. Roasted Veggie & Quinoa Bowls

Ingredient:

- 1 cup uncooked quinoa, rinsed
- 2 cups low•sodium vegetable or chicken broth
- 1 medium sweet potato, peeled and cubed
- 1 red bell pepper, chopped
- 1 zucchini, chopped
- 1 red onion, sliced
- 2 tbsp olive oil
- 1 tsp dried thyme
- 1 tsp dried oregano
- Salt and pepper to taste
- 4 cups baby spinach or kale
- 1/4 cup crumbled feta cheese (optional)
- 2 tbsp toasted pumpkin seeds (optional)

Dressing:
- 2 tbsp olive oil
- 1 tbsp balsamic vinegar
- 1 tbsp Dijon mustard
- 1 tsp honey
- Salt and pepper to taste

Instructions:

1. Preheat oven to 400°F. Line a large baking sheet with parchment paper.

2. In a medium saucepan, combine the quinoa and broth. Bring to a boil, then reduce heat and simmer for 15•20 minutes until quinoa is cooked. Fluff with a fork.

3. On the prepared baking sheet, toss the sweet potato, bell pepper, zucchini, and onion with 2 tbsp olive oil, thyme, oregano, salt and pepper. Roast for 20•25 minutes, stirring halfway, until veggies are tender.

4. In a small bowl, whisk together the dressing ingredients • 2 tbsp olive oil, balsamic vinegar, Dijon, honey, salt and pepper.

5. To assemble the bowls, divide the quinoa and roasted veggies among 4 serving bowls. Top each with 1 cup spinach/kale, 1 tbsp feta (if using), and 1.5 tsp toasted pumpkin seeds (if using). Drizzle the balsamic dressing over the top.

61. Zesty Lemon Chicken

Ingredient:

- 4 boneless, skinless chicken breasts
- 2 tbsp olive oil
- 2 tbsp freshly squeezed lemon juice
- 1 tbsp Dijon mustard
- 2 cloves garlic, minced
- 1 tsp dried oregano
- 1/2 tsp salt
- 1/4 tsp black pepper
- 1 lemon, thinly sliced (optional)
- Chopped parsley for garnish (optional)

Instructions:

1. In a shallow baking dish or resealable plastic bag, combine the olive oil, lemon juice, Dijon mustard, garlic, oregano, salt, and pepper. Add the chicken breasts and turn to coat them evenly in the marinade.

2. Cover the dish or seal the bag and refrigerate for 30 minutes to 1 hour, turning the chicken occasionally.

3. Preheat oven to 400°F.

4. Remove the chicken from the marinade and place in a baking dish. Arrange the lemon slices around the chicken, if using.

5. Bake for 20•25 minutes, until the chicken is cooked through and reaches an internal temperature of 165°F.

6. Remove the chicken from the oven and let it rest for 5 minutes.

7. Serve the Zesty Lemon Chicken warm, garnished with chopped parsley if desired. Drizzle any pan juices over the top.

This Zesty Lemon Chicken is a bright, flavorful, and healthy main dish. The lemon, Dijon, and garlic marinade gives the chicken a delicious zesty flavor. Serve it with your choice of sides like roasted vegetables or a fresh salad.

62. Chocolate Banana Protein Muffins

Ingredient:

- 1 cup mashed ripe bananas (about 2 medium bananas)
- 1/2 cup unsweetened applesauce
- 1/4 cup honey or maple syrup
- 2 large eggs
- 1 tsp vanilla extract
- 1 cup whole wheat flour
- 1/2 cup unflavored whey protein powder
- 1/4 cup unsweetened cocoa powder
- 1 tsp baking soda
- 1/4 tsp salt
- 1/2 cup dark chocolate chips (optional)

Instructions:

1. Preheat oven to 350°F. Grease a 12·cup muffin tin or line with paper liners.

2. In a large bowl, mash the bananas. Stir in the applesauce, honey/maple syrup, eggs, and vanilla until well combined.

3. In a separate bowl, whisk together the whole wheat flour, protein powder, cocoa powder, baking soda, and salt.

4. Fold the dry ingredients into the wet ingredients just until combined. Fold in the chocolate chips if using.

5. Divide the batter evenly among the prepared muffin cups, filling them about 3/4 full.

6. Bake for 18·22 minutes, until a toothpick inserted in the center comes out clean.

7. Allow the muffins to cool in the pan for 5 minutes before transferring to a wire rack to cool completely.

Enjoy these moist, chocolatey, protein·packed muffins! They make a great healthy snack or breakfast for both men and women.

63. Veggie·Packed Lentil Soup

Ingredient:

- 1 tbsp olive oil
- 1 onion, diced
- 3 carrots, peeled and diced
- 3 celery stalks, diced
- 3 cloves garlic, minced
- 1 tsp ground cumin
- 1 tsp dried oregano
- 1/2 tsp smoked paprika
- 1/4 tsp cayenne pepper (optional)
- 1 cup dry brown or green lentils, rinsed
- 6 cups low·sodium vegetable or chicken broth
- 1 (14.5 oz) can diced tomatoes
- 2 cups chopped kale or spinach
- 1 bay leaf
- Salt and pepper to taste
- Chopped parsley for garnish (optional)

Instructions:

1. In a large pot or Dutch oven, heat the olive oil over medium heat. Add the diced onion, carrots, and celery. Sauté for 5·7 minutes until softened.

2. Stir in the minced garlic, cumin, oregano, smoked paprika, and cayenne (if using). Cook for 1 minute until fragrant.

3. Add the rinsed lentils, broth, diced tomatoes, kale/spinach, and bay leaf. Season with salt and pepper.

4. Bring the soup to a boil, then reduce heat and let simmer for 25·30 minutes, until the lentils are tender.

5. Remove the bay leaf. Taste and adjust seasoning as needed.

6. Serve the Veggie·Packed Lentil Soup hot, garnished with chopped parsley if desired.

This hearty lentil soup is packed with fiber, protein, and nutrient·dense vegetables. It's a comforting and satisfying meal that both men and women will enjoy. Adjust the spice level to your preference.

64. Garlic Herb Grilled Chicken

Ingredient:

- 1.5 lbs boneless, skinless chicken breasts
- 3 tbsp olive oil
- 3 cloves garlic, minced
- 2 tsp dried oregano
- 1 tsp dried basil
- 1 tsp dried thyme
- 1 tsp salt
- 1/2 tsp black pepper

Marinade:

- 1/4 cup olive oil
- 2 tbsp lemon juice
- 2 tbsp low•sodium soy sauce
- 1 tbsp Dijon mustard
- 2 cloves garlic, minced
- 1 tsp dried oregano
- 1/2 tsp salt
- 1/4 tsp black pepper

Instructions:

1. In a small bowl, mix together the marinade ingredients • 1/4 cup olive oil, lemon juice, soy sauce, Dijon, 2 cloves minced garlic, 1 tsp oregano, 1/2 tsp salt, and 1/4 tsp pepper.

2. Place the chicken breasts in a resealable plastic bag or shallow baking dish. Pour the marinade over the chicken, turning to coat. Refrigerate for 30 minutes to 1 hour.

3. In another small bowl, combine the 3 tbsp olive oil, 3 cloves minced garlic, 2 tsp oregano, 1 tsp basil, 1 tsp thyme, 1 tsp salt, and 1/2 tsp pepper. Mix well.

4. Preheat grill to medium•high heat.

5. Remove the chicken from the marinade and discard the marinade. Brush the chicken all over with the garlic herb oil mixture.

6. Grill the chicken for 5•7 minutes per side, until cooked through and no longer pink in the center.

7. Let the chicken rest for 5 minutes before serving.

Serve the juicy, flavorful Garlic Herb Grilled Chicken with your choice of sides. This recipe is perfect for both men and women looking for a healthy, delicious grilled chicken dish.

65. Baked Avocado Fries

Ingredient:

- 2 ripe avocados, pitted and sliced into wedges
- 1/2 cup panko breadcrumbs
- 1/4 cup grated Parmesan cheese
- 1 tsp garlic powder
- 1/2 tsp paprika
- 1/4 tsp cayenne pepper (optional)
- Salt and pepper to taste
- 2 tbsp olive oil

Dipping Sauce (optional):
- 1/2 cup plain Greek yogurt
- 1 tbsp lime juice
- 1 tbsp chopped cilantro
- 1 tsp honey
- Salt and pepper to taste

Instructions:

1. Preheat oven to 400°F. Line a baking sheet with parchment paper.

2. In a shallow bowl, combine the panko, Parmesan, garlic powder, paprika, cayenne (if using), and a pinch of salt and pepper.

3. Gently toss the avocado wedges with the olive oil to lightly coat.

4. Working in batches, dredge the avocado wedges in the panko mixture, pressing gently to help it adhere.

5. Arrange the breaded avocado fries in a single layer on the prepared baking sheet.

6. Bake for 12·15 minutes, flipping halfway, until the fries are golden brown and crispy.

7. While the fries are baking, make the dipping sauce (if using). In a small bowl, mix together the Greek yogurt, lime juice, cilantro, honey, and a pinch of salt and pepper.

8. Serve the baked avocado fries immediately, with the dipping sauce on the side if desired.

66. Spicy Moroccan Chickpeas

Ingredient:

- 2 tbsp olive oil
- 1 onion, diced
- 3 cloves garlic, minced
- 1 tbsp grated fresh ginger
- 1 tsp ground cumin
- 1 tsp paprika
- 1 tsp ground coriander
- 1/2 tsp ground cinnamon
- 1/4 tsp cayenne pepper (or more to taste)
- 1 (15oz) can diced tomatoes
- 1 (15oz) can chickpeas, drained and rinsed
- 1 cup low•sodium vegetable or chicken broth
- 1 tsp honey
- Salt and pepper to taste
- Chopped cilantro for serving

Instructions:

1. In a large skillet or pot, heat the olive oil over medium heat. Add the diced onion and sauté for 5 minutes until translucent.

2. Add the minced garlic and grated ginger. Cook for 1 minute until fragrant.

3. Stir in the cumin, paprika, coriander, cinnamon, and cayenne. Cook for 1 minute to toast the spices.

4. Pour in the diced tomatoes, chickpeas, broth, and honey. Stir to combine.

5. Bring the mixture to a simmer and let cook for 10•15 minutes, until the sauce has thickened slightly. Season with salt and pepper to taste.

6. Remove from heat and stir in chopped fresh cilantro.Serve the spicy Moroccan chickpeas warm, over cooked quinoa, rice, or with pita bread.

This dish is packed with protein, fiber, and flavor from the aromatic Moroccan spices. It's a great vegetarian/vegan option that both men and women will enjoy. Adjust the spice level to your preference.

67. Lemon Poppy Seed Protein Muffins

Ingredient:

- 1 1/4 cups whole wheat flour
- 1/2 cup unflavored whey protein powder
- 1 tbsp poppy seeds
- 1 tsp baking powder
- 1/4 tsp baking soda
- 1/4 tsp salt
- 3 large eggs
- 1/2 cup plain Greek yogurt
- 1/4 cup honey
- 2 tbsp lemon juice
- 1 tbsp lemon zest
- 1 tsp vanilla extract

Instructions:

1. Preheat oven to 350°F. Grease a 12•cup muffin tin or line with paper liners.

2. In a medium bowl, whisk together the whole wheat flour, protein powder, poppy seeds, baking powder, baking soda, and salt.

3. In a separate large bowl, beat the eggs. Then stir in the Greek yogurt, honey, lemon juice, lemon zest, and vanilla until well combined.

4. Fold the dry ingredients into the wet ingredients just until combined, being careful not to overmix.

5. Divide the batter evenly among the prepared muffin cups, filling them about 3/4 full.

6. Bake for 16•18 minutes, until a toothpick inserted in the center comes out clean.

7. Allow the muffins to cool in the pan for 5 minutes before transferring to a wire rack to cool completely.

These Lemon Poppy Seed Protein Muffins are moist, flavorful, and packed with protein from the whey powder. They make a great healthy snack or breakfast for both men and women. Enjoy!

68. Beef & Broccoli Stir·Fry

Ingredient:

• 1 lb flank steak, thinly sliced against the grain
• 3 tbsp low·sodium soy sauce
• 2 tbsp rice vinegar
• 1 tbsp brown sugar
• 1 tsp sesame oil
• 2 cloves garlic, minced
• 1 tbsp grated fresh ginger
• 2 tbsp vegetable or canola oil
• 4 cups broccoli florets
• 1 red bell pepper, thinly sliced
• 2 green onions, sliced
• Cooked brown rice, for serving

Sauce:
• 2 tbsp low·sodium soy sauce
• 1 tbsp rice vinegar
• 1 tsp cornstarch
• 1/4 tsp red pepper flakes (optional)

Instructions:

1. In a medium bowl, combine the sliced beef, 3 tbsp soy sauce, 2 tbsp rice vinegar, brown sugar, and sesame oil. Toss to coat and let marinate for 15·30 minutes.

2. In a small bowl, whisk together the sauce ingredients • 2 tbsp soy sauce, 1 tbsp rice vinegar, cornstarch, and red pepper flakes if using. Set aside.

3. Heat 1 tbsp of the vegetable oil in a large skillet or wok over high heat. Add the beef and marinade and stir·fry for 2·3 minutes until beef is browned. Remove beef from pan and set aside.

4. Add the remaining 1 tbsp oil to the pan. Add the broccoli and bell pepper and stir·fry for 3·4 minutes until crisp·tender.

5. Return the beef and any accumulated juices to the pan. Pour in the sauce and toss everything together, cooking for 1·2 minutes until the sauce has thickened.

6. Remove from heat and stir in the green onions.. Serve the beef and broccoli stir·fry immediately over cooked brown rice.

69. Buffalo Chicken Stuffed Peppers

Ingredient:

- 6 bell peppers, halved lengthwise and seeds removed
- 1 lb boneless, skinless chicken breasts, cooked and shredded
- 1/2 cup hot sauce (such as Frank's RedHot)
- 1/2 cup crumbled blue cheese
- 1/2 cup shredded cheddar cheese
- 1/4 cup diced celery
- 2 tbsp ranch dressing
- Salt and pepper to taste

Instructions:

1. Preheat oven to 375°F. Arrange the bell pepper halves cut·side up in a baking dish.

2. In a large bowl, mix together the shredded chicken, hot sauce, blue cheese, cheddar cheese, celery and ranch dressing. Season with salt and pepper.

3. Spoon the buffalo chicken mixture evenly into the bell pepper halves, packing it in tightly.

4. Bake for 20·25 minutes, until the peppers are tender and the filling is hot and bubbly.

5. Serve the buffalo chicken stuffed peppers immediately, garnished with extra blue cheese crumbles and chopped green onions if desired.

This recipe is great for both men and women because:

- It's high in protein from the chicken
- The buffalo flavor provides a tasty kick
- The bell peppers add a nice crunch and nutrition
- It's easy to prepare with simple, wholesome ingredients
- It can be customized to individual taste preferences (e.g. adjust hot sauce amount)

The combination of bold buffalo flavor, melty cheeses, and tender bell peppers makes this a satisfying and nutritious meal option. Enjoy!

70. Roasted Beet & Quinoa Salad

Ingredient:

- 3 medium beets, peeled and cut into 1·inch cubes
- 2 tbsp olive oil
- Salt and pepper to taste
- 1 cup uncooked quinoa, rinsed
- 2 cups vegetable or chicken broth
- 1 cup crumbled feta cheese
- 1/4 cup chopped fresh parsley
- 2 tbsp balsamic vinegar
- 1 tbsp honey
- 1 tsp Dijon mustard

Instructions:

1. Preheat oven to 400°F. Toss the cubed beets with 1 tbsp olive oil and season with salt and pepper. Spread on a baking sheet and roast for 20·25 minutes, until tender. Let cool slightly.

2. In a medium saucepan, combine the quinoa and broth. Bring to a boil, then reduce heat to low, cover and simmer for 15·20 minutes, until quinoa is cooked through. Fluff with a fork and let cool.

3. In a large bowl, combine the roasted beets, cooked quinoa, feta cheese and parsley.

4. In a small bowl, whisk together the remaining 1 tbsp olive oil, balsamic vinegar, honey and Dijon mustard. Season with salt and pepper.

5. Drizzle the dressing over the salad and toss gently to coat. Serve immediately or refrigerate until ready to serve.

Enjoy this colorful and nutritious beet and quinoa salad! Let me know if you have any other questions.

71. Teriyaki Chicken Bowls

Ingredient:

Teriyaki Chicken:
• 1 lb boneless, skinless chicken breasts, cut into 1•inch pieces
• 1/4 cup low•sodium soy sauce
• 2 tbsp brown sugar
• 2 tbsp rice vinegar
• 1 tbsp sesame oil
• 2 cloves garlic, minced
• 1 tsp grated fresh ginger

Bowls:
• 2 cups cooked brown rice
• 1 cup shredded carrots
• 1 cup thinly sliced cucumber
• 1/2 cup thinly sliced green onions
• 2 tbsp toasted sesame seeds
• Chopped cilantro for garnish (optional)

Instructions:

1. In a medium bowl, whisk together the soy sauce, brown sugar, rice vinegar, sesame oil, garlic, and ginger. Add the chicken pieces and toss to coat. Cover and marinate for 30 minutes to 1 hour.

2. Heat a large skillet or wok over medium•high heat. Add the marinated chicken and cook for 5•7 minutes, stirring occasionally, until the chicken is cooked through.

3. To assemble the bowls, divide the cooked brown rice among 4 serving bowls. Top each with some of the cooked teriyaki chicken, shredded carrots, sliced cucumber, green onions, and toasted sesame seeds.

4. Garnish with chopped cilantro if desired.

5. Serve the Teriyaki Chicken Bowls immediately, while the chicken is hot.

These Teriyaki Chicken Bowls are a delicious and nutritious meal that both men and women will enjoy. The flavorful teriyaki chicken pairs perfectly with the fresh veggies and nutty brown rice. Adjust the portion sizes as needed to suit your dietary needs.

72. Almond·Crusted Salmon

Ingredient:

- 4 salmon fillets (about 6 oz each)
- 1/2 cup sliced almonds
- 2 tbsp panko breadcrumbs
- 2 tbsp grated Parmesan cheese
- 1 tbsp olive oil
- 1 tsp lemon zest
- 1/4 tsp salt
- 1/4 tsp black pepper

Instructions:

1. Preheat oven to 400°F. Line a baking sheet with parchment paper.

2. In a shallow bowl, combine the sliced almonds, panko breadcrumbs, Parmesan cheese, olive oil, lemon zest, salt and pepper. Mix well.

3. Place the salmon fillets skin·side down on the prepared baking sheet. Gently press the almond mixture onto the top of each salmon fillet, covering the surface completely.

4. Bake for 12·15 minutes, until the salmon is cooked through and the almond crust is golden brown.

5. Serve the almond·crusted salmon immediately, garnished with lemon wedges if desired.

This recipe is a great option for both men and women as it is:

- High in protein from the salmon
- Provides healthy fats from the almonds
- Packed with flavor from the Parmesan, lemon and spices
- Easy to prepare with simple, wholesome ingredients

The almond crust adds a nice crunch and nutty flavor to the salmon, making it an elegant yet easy·to·prepare main dish. Enjoy!

73. Baked Sweet Potato Chips

Ingredient:

- 2 medium sweet potatoes, peeled and sliced into 1/8•inch thick rounds
- 2 tbsp olive oil
- 1 tsp paprika
- 1/2 tsp garlic powder
- 1/2 tsp salt
- 1/4 tsp black pepper

Instructions:

1. Preheat oven to 400°F. Line two baking sheets with parchment paper.

2. In a large bowl, toss the sweet potato slices with the olive oil, paprika, garlic powder, salt and pepper until evenly coated.

3. Arrange the sweet potato slices in a single layer on the prepared baking sheets, making sure they don't overlap.

4. Bake for 15•20 minutes, flipping the chips halfway through, until lightly browned and crispy.

5. Remove the baked sweet potato chips from the oven and let cool completely before serving.

These baked sweet potato chips make a delicious and healthy snack or side dish. The simple seasoning of paprika, garlic, salt and pepper adds great flavor without a lot of extra calories or fat. Sweet potatoes are packed with vitamins, minerals and fiber, making these chips a nutritious alternative to regular potato chips.

Enjoy these crispy, flavorful baked sweet potato chips! Let me know if you have any other questions.

74. Spicy Turkey & Veggie Skillet

Ingredient:

- 2 medium sweet potatoes, peeled and sliced into 1/8•inch thick rounds
- 2 tbsp olive oil
- 1 tsp paprika
- 1/2 tsp garlic powder
- 1/2 tsp salt
- 1/4 tsp black pepper

Instructions:

1. Preheat oven to 400°F. Line two baking sheets with parchment paper.

2. In a large bowl, toss the sweet potato slices with the olive oil, paprika, garlic powder, salt and pepper until evenly coated.

3. Arrange the sweet potato slices in a single layer on the prepared baking sheets, making sure they don't overlap.

4. Bake for 15•20 minutes, flipping the chips halfway through, until lightly browned and crispy.

5. Remove the baked sweet potato chips from the oven and let cool completely before serving.

This recipe is great for both men and women because:

- Sweet potatoes are a nutritious, complex carbohydrate that provides fiber, vitamins, and minerals

- The baking method makes these chips a healthier alternative to fried potato chips

- The simple seasoning of paprika, garlic, salt and pepper adds flavor without a lot of extra calories or fat

- Sweet potato chips are a satisfying, crunchy snack that can be enjoyed by people of all ages and dietary preferences

Baked sweet potato chips are a versatile, nutrient•dense snack that can be enjoyed by both men and women as part of a balanced, healthy diet. Enjoy!

75. Garlic Parmesan Roasted Cauliflower

Ingredient:

- 1 head of cauliflower, cut into florets
- 3 tbsp olive oil
- 3 cloves garlic, minced
- 1/2 cup grated Parmesan cheese
- 1 tsp dried parsley
- 1/2 tsp salt
- 1/4 tsp black pepper

Instructions:

1. Preheat oven to 400°F. Line a large baking sheet with parchment paper.

2. In a large bowl, toss the cauliflower florets with the olive oil and garlic until evenly coated.

3. Spread the cauliflower in a single layer on the prepared baking sheet.

4. In a small bowl, mix together the Parmesan cheese, dried parsley, salt and pepper.

5. Sprinkle the Parmesan cheese mixture evenly over the cauliflower.

6. Roast for 20•25 minutes, stirring halfway, until the cauliflower is tender and the Parmesan is golden brown.

7. Serve the garlic Parmesan roasted cauliflower immediately, garnished with extra parsley if desired.

This recipe is great for both men and women because:

- Cauliflower is a nutrient•dense vegetable packed with vitamins, minerals and fiber
- The Parmesan cheese and garlic add savory, umami flavors without a lot of extra calories
- Roasting brings out the natural sweetness of the cauliflower
- It's a simple, easy•to•prepare side dish that complements a variety of main courses

Garlic Parmesan roasted cauliflower is a delicious and healthy option that can be enjoyed by both men and women as part of a balanced diet. Enjoy!

76. Grilled Chicken & Veggie Kabobs

Ingredient:

- 1 lb boneless, skinless chicken breasts, cut into 1•inch cubes
- 1 red bell pepper, cut into 1•inch pieces
- 1 yellow bell pepper, cut into 1•inch pieces
- 1 zucchini, cut into 1•inch rounds
- 1 red onion, cut into 1•inch pieces
- 8 oz mushrooms, halved
- 2 tbsp olive oil
- 2 tbsp balsamic vinegar
- 1 tsp dried oregano
- 1 tsp garlic powder
- Salt and pepper to taste
- Wooden or metal skewers

Instructions:

1. In a large bowl, combine the chicken, bell peppers, zucchini, onion, and mushrooms.

2. In a small bowl, whisk together the olive oil, balsamic vinegar, oregano, garlic powder, salt, and pepper.

3. Pour the marinade over the chicken and vegetables and toss to coat evenly. Cover and refrigerate for 30 minutes to 1 hour.

4. Preheat grill to medium•high heat.

5. Thread the marinated chicken and vegetables onto the skewers, alternating the ingredients.

6. Grill the kabobs for 12•15 minutes, turning occasionally, until the chicken is cooked through and the vegetables are tender. Serve the grilled chicken and veggie kabobs immediately.

This recipe is great for both men and women because:

- It's high in protein from the chicken
- The vegetables provide a variety of vitamins, minerals, and fiber
- The marinade adds flavor without a lot of extra calories or fat
- Grilling is a healthy cooking method that retains nutrients
- It's a complete, balanced meal that can be easily customized to individual tastes

77. Spinach & Mushroom Stuffed Peppers

Ingredient:

- 6 bell peppers, halved lengthwise and seeds removed
- 1 tbsp olive oil
- 8 oz mushrooms, sliced
- 1 onion, diced
- 3 cloves garlic, minced
- 5 oz baby spinach, chopped
- 1 cup cooked brown rice
- 1/2 cup crumbled feta cheese
- 1/4 cup grated Parmesan cheese
- 1 tsp dried oregano
- Salt and pepper to taste

Instructions:

1. Preheat oven to 375°F. Arrange the bell pepper halves cut•side up in a baking dish.

2. In a large skillet, heat the olive oil over medium heat. Add the mushrooms and onion, and sauté for 5•7 minutes until softened.

3. Add the garlic and spinach to the skillet. Cook for 2•3 minutes, stirring frequently, until the spinach is wilted. Remove from heat.

4. In a bowl, mix together the sautéed mushroom•spinach mixture, cooked brown rice, feta cheese, Parmesan cheese, and oregano. Season with salt and pepper.

5. Spoon the spinach and mushroom filling evenly into the bell pepper halves.

6. Bake for 20•25 minutes, until the peppers are tender and the filling is hot.

7. Serve the stuffed peppers warm, garnished with extra Parmesan cheese if desired.

These spinach and mushroom stuffed peppers make a delicious and nutritious meal. The combination of the tender bell peppers, savory filling, and melty cheeses creates a satisfying dish. Enjoy!

78. BBQ Chicken Flatbread

Ingredient:

- 1 lb boneless, skinless chicken breasts
- 1 cup barbecue sauce, divided
- 1 pre•baked flatbread or naan
- 1 cup shredded mozzarella cheese
- 1/2 red onion, thinly sliced
- 2 tbsp chopped fresh cilantro

Instructions:

1. Preheat oven to 400°F.

2. Place the chicken breasts in a baking dish and brush with 1/4 cup of the barbecue sauce. Bake for 20•25 minutes, until the chicken is cooked through. Shred or chop the cooked chicken.

3. Spread the remaining 3/4 cup of barbecue sauce evenly over the flatbread or naan.

4. Top the flatbread with the shredded chicken, mozzarella cheese, and sliced red onion.

5. Bake for 10•12 minutes, until the cheese is melted and bubbly.

6. Remove the BBQ chicken flatbread from the oven and sprinkle with the chopped fresh cilantro.

7. Slice and serve immediately.

This BBQ chicken flatbread makes a delicious and easy•to•prepare meal or appetizer. The combination of the tangy barbecue sauce, tender chicken, melty cheese, and fresh onion and cilantro creates a flavorful and satisfying dish. Enjoy!

79. Protein·Packed Smoothie Bowl

Ingredient:

• 1 cup unsweetened almond milk
• 1 scoop vanilla protein powder
• 1 frozen banana
• 1/2 cup frozen mixed berries
• 2 tbsp almond butter
• 1 tbsp chia seeds
• 1 tbsp hemp seeds
• Toppings: sliced banana, berries, granola, shredded coconut, etc.

Instructions:

1. In a high·powered blender, combine the almond milk, protein powder, frozen banana, frozen berries, and almond butter. Blend until smooth and creamy.

2. Pour the smoothie into a bowl.

3. Top the smoothie bowl with your desired toppings such as sliced banana, fresh berries, granola, shredded coconut, etc.

This protein·packed smoothie bowl is a great option for both men and women for several reasons:

• Protein from the protein powder helps build and maintain muscle mass
• Healthy fats from the almond butter and seeds provide sustained energy
• Fiber and antioxidants from the fruits and vegetables support overall health
• The thick, creamy texture makes it filling and satisfying
• It can be customized with different protein powders, fruits, and toppings to suit individual tastes

The combination of protein, healthy fats, fiber, and nutrients makes this smoothie bowl a nutritious and balanced meal or snack. It's a great way to start the day or refuel after a workout.

Enjoy this delicious and nourishing protein·packed smoothie bowl!

80. Chicken & Avocado Salad

Ingredient:

- 2 cups cooked, shredded chicken
- 1 avocado, diced
- 1/2 cup diced celery
- 1/4 cup diced red onion
- 2 tbsp chopped fresh cilantro
- 2 tbsp olive oil
- 1 tbsp lime juice
- 1 tsp Dijon mustard
- Salt and pepper to taste

Instructions:

1. In a large bowl, combine the shredded chicken, diced avocado, celery, red onion, and chopped cilantro.

2. In a small bowl, whisk together the olive oil, lime juice, and Dijon mustard. Season with salt and pepper.

3. Pour the dressing over the chicken and avocado mixture and toss gently to coat.

4. Serve the chicken and avocado salad chilled or at room temperature. It can be served on its own, on a bed of greens, or with crackers or bread.

This chicken and avocado salad is a delicious and nutritious option that's perfect for a light lunch or snack. The combination of lean protein from the chicken, healthy fats from the avocado, and crunchy vegetables makes it a satisfying and well·balanced meal.

Some of the benefits of this recipe include:

- High in protein and healthy fats to keep you feeling full and satisfied
- Packed with vitamins, minerals, and antioxidants from the avocado, celery, and cilantro
- Easy to prepare with simple, fresh ingredients
- Versatile · can be served in a variety of ways

Enjoy this tasty and nutritious chicken and avocado salad!

81. Zucchini Noodle Pad Thai

Ingredient:

- 3 medium zucchinis, spiralized or julienned into noodles
- 8 oz cooked shrimp or chicken, chopped
- 2 tbsp peanut oil
- 2 cloves garlic, minced
- 1 egg, lightly beaten
- 2 tbsp fish sauce
- 2 tbsp lime juice
- 1 tbsp brown sugar
- 1 tsp Sriracha or other hot sauce (optional)
- 2 tbsp chopped roasted peanuts
- 2 tbsp chopped fresh cilantro
- 1 lime, cut into wedges for serving

Instructions:

1. In a large skillet or wok, heat the peanut oil over medium•high heat. Add the garlic and cook for 1 minute until fragrant.

2. Add the zucchini noodles and shrimp/chicken to the skillet. Stir•fry for 2•3 minutes until the zucchini is tender•crisp.

3. Push the noodle mixture to the side of the pan. Pour the beaten egg into the empty side and let it cook for 1 minute, then scramble it into the noodles.

4. In a small bowl, whisk together the fish sauce, lime juice, brown sugar, and Sriracha (if using).

5. Add the sauce to the skillet and toss everything together until well coated and heated through, about 2 more minutes.

6. Remove from heat and stir in the chopped peanuts and cilantro.. Serve the zucchini noodle pad thai immediately, with lime wedges on the side.

This zucchini noodle pad thai is a lighter, veggie•packed version of the classic Thai dish. It's a great option for both men and women as it's:

- High in protein from the shrimp/chicken
- Packed with nutrients from the zucchini noodles and other veggies
- Flavorful from the Thai•inspired sauce
- Easy to prepare and customize to your taste preference

84. Buffalo Turkey Meatballs

Ingredient:

- 1 lb ground turkey
- 1/2 cup panko breadcrumbs
- 1/4 cup crumbled blue cheese
- 2 tbsp chopped fresh parsley
- 1 egg, lightly beaten
- 1/2 tsp garlic powder
- 1/4 tsp cayenne pepper
- 1/4 tsp salt
- 1/4 tsp black pepper
- 1/2 cup buffalo sauce (such as Frank's RedHot)
- 2 tbsp ranch or blue cheese dressing (optional)

Instructions:

1. Preheat oven to 400°F. Line a baking sheet with parchment paper.

2. In a large bowl, combine the ground turkey, panko, blue cheese, parsley, egg, garlic powder, cayenne, salt, and pepper. Mix until just combined, being careful not to overmix.

3. Roll the mixture into 1•inch meatballs and place them on the prepared baking sheet.

4. Bake for 18•20 minutes, until the meatballs are cooked through.

5. In a large bowl, toss the baked meatballs with the buffalo sauce until evenly coated.

6. Serve the buffalo turkey meatballs warm, with ranch or blue cheese dressing for dipping, if desired.

The combination of tender, juicy turkey meatballs and the spicy buffalo sauce makes these a delicious and nutritious option that can be enjoyed by both men and women. Enjoy!

85. Teriyaki Beef Skewers

Ingredient:

- 1 lb beef sirloin or flank steak, cut into 1·inch cubes
- 1/2 cup teriyaki sauce
- 2 tbsp brown sugar
- 2 cloves garlic, minced
- 1 tsp grated fresh ginger
- 1/4 tsp red pepper flakes (optional)
- Wooden or metal skewers

Instructions:

1. In a large resealable bag or bowl, combine the beef cubes, teriyaki sauce, brown sugar, garlic, ginger, and red pepper flakes (if using). Toss to coat the beef evenly. Cover and marinate in the refrigerator for at least 30 minutes, up to 4 hours.

2. Preheat grill or grill pan to medium·high heat.

3. Thread the marinated beef cubes onto the skewers, leaving a small space between each piece.

4. Grill the beef skewers for 2·3 minutes per side, or until cooked to your desired doneness.

5. Serve the teriyaki beef skewers immediately, garnished with chopped green onions or sesame seeds if desired.

These teriyaki beef skewers are a great option for both men and women for a few reasons:

- Beef is a good source of protein, which is important for building and maintaining muscle mass.
- The teriyaki marinade adds flavor without a lot of extra calories or fat.
- Grilling is a healthy cooking method that retains nutrients.
- The skewers are easy to prepare and make a fun, portable meal or appetizer.
- The dish can be customized by adjusting the amount of heat from the red pepper flakes.

The combination of tender, flavorful beef and the sweet and savory teriyaki glaze makes these skewers a crowd·pleasing option for both men and women. Enjoy!

88. Spicy Chickpea & Veggie Tacos

Ingredient:

- 1 (15 oz) can chickpeas, drained and rinsed
- 1 tbsp olive oil
- 1 tsp chili powder
- 1/2 tsp cumin
- 1/4 tsp cayenne pepper (or more to taste)
- Salt and pepper to taste
- 1 cup shredded red cabbage
- 1 cup diced tomatoes
- 1/2 cup diced avocado
- 1/4 cup chopped fresh cilantro
- 8•10 small corn or flour tortillas
- Lime wedges for serving

Instructions:

1. In a medium skillet, heat the olive oil over medium heat. Add the chickpeas and season with the chili powder, cumin, cayenne, salt, and pepper. Cook for 5•7 minutes, stirring occasionally, until the chickpeas are lightly crispy.

2. In a bowl, combine the shredded red cabbage, diced tomatoes, diced avocado, and chopped cilantro.

3. To assemble the tacos, place a spoonful of the spicy chickpeas into each tortilla. Top with the veggie mixture.

4. Serve the spicy chickpea and veggie tacos immediately, with lime wedges on the side for squeezing over the top.

These spicy chickpea and veggie tacos make a delicious, nutritious, and easy•to•prepare meal. Some of the benefits include:

- Chickpeas provide plant•based protein and fiber
- The vegetables add vitamins, minerals, and antioxidants
- The spices add bold flavor without a lot of extra calories or fat
- It's a versatile dish that can be customized to individual tastes
- Tacos are a fun, handheld way to enjoy a balanced meal

Enjoy these flavorful and satisfying spicy chickpea and veggie tacos!

89. Maple Cinnamon Roasted Sweet Potatoes

Ingredient:

- 3 medium sweet potatoes, peeled and cut into 1·inch cubes
- 2 tbsp olive oil
- 2 tbsp pure maple syrup
- 1 tsp ground cinnamon
- 1/4 tsp ground nutmeg
- 1/4 tsp salt
- 1/8 tsp black pepper

Instructions:

1. Preheat oven to 400°F. Line a large baking sheet with parchment paper.

2. In a large bowl, toss the sweet potato cubes with the olive oil, maple syrup, cinnamon, nutmeg, salt, and pepper until evenly coated.

3. Spread the seasoned sweet potato cubes in a single layer on the prepared baking sheet.

4. Roast for 25·30 minutes, flipping the potatoes halfway through, until they are tender and lightly caramelized.

5. Remove the roasted sweet potatoes from the oven and transfer to a serving dish.

6. Serve the maple cinnamon roasted sweet potatoes warm.

These maple cinnamon roasted sweet potatoes make a delicious and healthy side dish. The natural sweetness of the sweet potatoes is enhanced by the maple syrup, while the cinnamon and nutmeg add warmth and depth of flavor.

Some benefits of this recipe:

- Sweet potatoes are an excellent source of vitamins, minerals, and antioxidants
- The maple syrup provides natural sweetness without refined sugar
- Roasting brings out the natural sugars in the sweet potatoes
- The simple seasoning complements the sweet potato flavor without overpowering it

92. Chicken & Veggie Stir·Fry

Ingredient:

- 1 lb boneless, skinless chicken breasts, cut into 1·inch pieces
- 2 tbsp sesame oil
- 3 cloves garlic, minced
- 1 tbsp grated fresh ginger
- 1 red bell pepper, sliced
- 1 cup broccoli florets
- 1 cup snow peas
- 1/2 cup sliced mushrooms
- 2 tbsp low·sodium soy sauce
- 1 tbsp rice vinegar
- 1 tsp cornstarch
- Salt and pepper to taste
- Cooked brown rice, for serving

Instructions:

1. In a large skillet or wok, heat the sesame oil over high heat. Add the chicken and cook for 3·4 minutes, until lightly browned.

2. Add the garlic and ginger to the skillet and cook for 1 minute, until fragrant.

3. Add the bell pepper, broccoli, snow peas, and mushrooms to the skillet. Stir·fry for 4·5 minutes, until the vegetables are tender·crisp.

4. In a small bowl, whisk together the soy sauce, rice vinegar, and cornstarch. Pour the sauce into the skillet and toss everything together until the sauce thickens, about 1·2 minutes.

5. Season the chicken and veggie stir·fry with salt and pepper to taste.

6. Serve the stir·fry immediately over cooked brown rice.

This chicken and veggie stir·fry is a great option for both men and women for several reasons:

- It's high in protein from the chicken, which helps build and maintain muscle mass.
- The variety of vegetables provides fiber, vitamins, minerals, and antioxidants.
- The ginger, garlic, and soy sauce add bold, savory flavors without a lot of extra calories or fat.

93. Balsamic Glazed Chicken

Ingredient:

- 4 boneless, skinless chicken breasts
- 2 tbsp olive oil
- 1/2 cup balsamic vinegar
- 2 tbsp honey
- 2 cloves garlic, minced
- 1 tsp dried thyme
- 1/4 tsp salt
- 1/4 tsp black pepper

Instructions:

1. Preheat oven to 400°F. Lightly grease a baking dish or line with parchment paper.

2. In a shallow bowl, whisk together the balsamic vinegar, honey, garlic, thyme, salt, and pepper.

3. Add the chicken breasts to the balsamic mixture and turn to coat both sides.

4. Place the chicken in the prepared baking dish. Pour any remaining balsamic mixture over the top.

5. Bake for 25•30 minutes, basting the chicken with the glaze halfway through, until the chicken is cooked through and the glaze is thickened.

6. Remove the balsamic glazed chicken from the oven and let rest for 5 minutes.

7. Serve the chicken warm, drizzled with any remaining glaze from the baking dish.

This balsamic glazed chicken is a great option for both men and women for a few reasons:

- Chicken is a lean protein that is high in protein and low in fat.
- The balsamic vinegar and honey create a sweet and tangy glaze that adds tons of flavor.
- The simple seasoning of garlic and thyme complements the balsamic without overpowering it.
- Baking is a healthy cooking method that retains the chicken's moisture and nutrients.

96. Spicy Sriracha Shrimp

Ingredient:

- 1 lb large shrimp, peeled and deveined
- 2 tbsp olive oil
- 2 tbsp Sriracha hot sauce
- 1 tbsp honey
- 2 cloves garlic, minced
- 1 tsp lime juice
- 1/4 tsp salt
- 1/4 tsp black pepper
- Chopped fresh cilantro for garnish (optional)

Instructions:

1. In a large bowl, combine the shrimp, olive oil, Sriracha, honey, garlic, lime juice, salt, and pepper. Toss to coat the shrimp evenly.

2. Heat a large skillet or wok over medium•high heat.

3. Add the marinated shrimp to the hot skillet and cook for 2•3 minutes per side, until the shrimp are opaque and cooked through.

4. Remove the spicy sriracha shrimp from the heat.

5. Serve the shrimp immediately, garnished with chopped fresh cilantro if desired. Enjoy with steamed rice, quinoa, or a fresh salad.

This spicy sriracha shrimp recipe is great for both men and women for a few reasons:

- Shrimp is a lean protein that is high in protein and low in fat.
- The Sriracha and honey create a bold, flavorful glaze that adds heat and sweetness.
- The quick cooking method preserves the natural texture and nutrients of the shrimp.
- It's an easy, one•pan dish that can be prepared in under 20 minutes.
- The dish can be customized to individual spice preferences by adjusting the amount of Sriracha.

The combination of tender, juicy shrimp and the spicy•sweet sriracha glaze makes this an appetizing and nutritious option that can be enjoyed by both men and women. Enjoy!

97. Pesto Chicken & Veggie Bowl

Ingredient:

- 1 lb boneless, skinless chicken breasts, grilled and sliced
- 2 cups cooked quinoa
- 1 cup cherry tomatoes, halved
- 1 cup steamed broccoli florets
- 1/2 cup roasted red peppers, sliced
- 1/4 cup basil pesto
- 2 tbsp toasted pine nuts
- 2 tbsp grated Parmesan cheese
- Salt and pepper to taste

Instructions:

1. Grill or bake the chicken breasts until cooked through. Slice or chop the chicken into bite•sized pieces.

2. In a large bowl, combine the cooked quinoa, sliced chicken, cherry tomatoes, steamed broccoli, and roasted red pepper slices.

3. Drizzle the basil pesto over the bowl and gently toss to coat the ingredients.

4. Top the pesto chicken and veggie bowl with the toasted pine nuts and grated Parmesan cheese.

5. Season with salt and pepper to taste. Serve the pesto chicken and veggie bowl immediately, while warm.

This recipe is great for both men and women because:

- It's high in protein from the grilled chicken
- The quinoa and vegetables provide complex carbs, fiber, vitamins, and minerals
- The basil pesto adds a flavorful, nutrient•dense sauce
- The pine nuts and Parmesan provide healthy fats and extra flavor
- It's a complete, balanced meal that can be easily customized

The combination of tender chicken, fluffy quinoa, fresh veggies, and vibrant pesto makes this a delicious and nutritious option that can be enjoyed by both men and women. It's a great way to get a variety of nutrients in one satisfying bowl.

Enjoy this pesto chicken and veggie bowl!

100. Spicy Black Bean & Sweet Potato Tacos

Ingredient:

- 2 medium sweet potatoes, peeled and diced
- 1 tbsp olive oil
- 1 tsp chili powder
- 1/2 tsp cumin
- Salt and pepper to taste
- 1 (15 oz) can black beans, drained and rinsed
- 1 jalapeño, seeded and minced
- 2 cloves garlic, minced
- 1 tsp lime juice
- 8·10 small corn or flour tortillas
- Toppings: shredded cabbage, diced avocado, crumbled queso fresco, chopped cilantro, lime wedges

Instructions:

1. Preheat oven to 400°F (200°C). Toss the diced sweet potatoes with the olive oil, chili powder, cumin, salt and pepper. Spread on a baking sheet and roast for 20·25 minutes, until tender.

2. In a skillet, sauté the jalapeño and garlic over medium heat for 1·2 minutes until fragrant. Add the black beans and lime juice. Mash some of the beans with a fork or potato masher to create a slightly chunky texture. Season with salt and pepper.

3. To assemble the tacos, warm the tortillas according to package instructions. Top each tortilla with some of the roasted sweet potatoes, black bean mixture, and desired toppings.

4. Serve the tacos immediately, with extra lime wedges on the side.

Enjoy your Spicy Black Bean & Sweet Potato Tacos! The combination of the sweet potatoes, spicy black beans, and fresh toppings makes for a delicious and nutritious vegetarian taco.

101. Ginger Garlic Grilled Chicken

Ingredient:

- 1.5 lbs boneless, skinless chicken breasts
- 3 cloves garlic, minced
- 1 tbsp freshly grated ginger
- 2 tbsp low•sodium soy sauce
- 1 tbsp rice vinegar
- 1 tbsp honey
- 1 tsp sesame oil
- 1/4 tsp red pepper flakes (optional, for spice)
- Salt and pepper to taste

Instructions:

1. In a large resealable bag or shallow baking dish, combine the minced garlic, grated ginger, soy sauce, rice vinegar, honey, sesame oil, and red pepper flakes (if using). Season with salt and pepper.

2. Add the chicken breasts to the marinade and turn to coat evenly. Cover and refrigerate for at least 30 minutes, up to 4 hours.

3. Preheat grill or grill pan to medium•high heat.

4. Remove the chicken from the marinade and discard any remaining marinade.

5. Grill the chicken for 5•7 minutes per side, or until cooked through and no longer pink in the center. The internal temperature should reach 165°F (75°C).

6. Transfer the grilled chicken to a cutting board and let rest for 5 minutes before slicing or serving.

Serve the Ginger Garlic Grilled Chicken with your choice of sides, such as roasted vegetables, rice, or a fresh salad. This recipe is a great option for a healthy, flavorful meal that both men and women can enjoy.

104. Lemon Herb Roasted Salmon

Ingredient:

- 1.5 lbs salmon fillets, skin•on or skinless
- 2 tbsp olive oil
- 2 tbsp freshly squeezed lemon juice
- 2 tsp lemon zest
- 2 cloves garlic, minced
- 1 tbsp chopped fresh dill
- 1 tbsp chopped fresh parsley
- 1/2 tsp salt
- 1/4 tsp black pepper

Instructions:

1. Preheat your oven to 400°F (200°C). Line a baking sheet with parchment paper or foil.

2. In a small bowl, whisk together the olive oil, lemon juice, lemon zest, garlic, dill, parsley, salt, and pepper.

3. Place the salmon fillets, skin•side down if using skin•on, on the prepared baking sheet. Spoon the lemon•herb mixture evenly over the top of the salmon.

4. Roast the salmon in the preheated oven for 12•15 minutes, or until it flakes easily with a fork and reaches an internal temperature of 145°F (63°C).

5. Serve the Lemon Herb Roasted Salmon immediately, garnished with additional fresh dill or parsley if desired. Enjoy!

This recipe is a simple and flavorful way to prepare salmon. The lemon, garlic, and fresh herbs complement the rich, omega•3•packed salmon perfectly. Serve it with roasted vegetables, a salad, or your favorite side dish for a healthy and delicious meal.

105. BBQ Beef & Veggie Skillet

Ingredient:

- 1 lb ground beef
- 1 onion, diced
- 2 cloves garlic, minced
- 1 bell pepper, diced
- 1 cup sliced mushrooms
- 1 cup diced zucchini
- 1 cup diced tomatoes (or 1 (14 oz) can diced tomatoes)
- 1/2 cup barbecue sauce
- 1 tsp chili powder
- 1/2 tsp smoked paprika
- Salt and pepper to taste
- Chopped fresh parsley for garnish (optional)

Instructions:

1. In a large skillet or cast•iron pan, cook the ground beef over medium•high heat, breaking it up with a wooden spoon, until browned and cooked through, about 5•7 minutes. Drain any excess fat.

2. Add the diced onion and minced garlic to the skillet. Sauté for 2•3 minutes until the onion is translucent.

3. Stir in the diced bell pepper, sliced mushrooms, and diced zucchini. Cook for 5•7 minutes, until the vegetables are tender.

4. Pour in the diced tomatoes (with their juices) and the barbecue sauce. Add the chili powder, smoked paprika, and season with salt and pepper to taste.

5. Bring the mixture to a simmer and let it cook for 10•15 minutes, stirring occasionally, until the sauce has thickened and the flavors have melded.

6. Serve the BBQ Beef & Veggie Skillet hot, garnished with chopped fresh parsley if desired.

This one•pan skillet dish is a great way to pack in a variety of vegetables and lean protein. The barbecue sauce and spices give it a delicious, bold flavor. Serve it on its own or with rice, quinoa, or a side salad for a complete and satisfying meal.

106. Spicy Turkey & Black Bean Chili

Ingredient:

- 1 lb ground turkey
- 1 tbsp olive oil
- 1 onion, diced
- 3 cloves garlic, minced
- 2 jalapeños, seeded and diced
- 2 tbsp chili powder
- 1 tsp cumin
- 1 tsp oregano
- 1/2 tsp smoked paprika
- 1/4 tsp cayenne pepper (optional, for extra heat)
- 1 (15 oz) can black beans, drained and rinsed
- 1 (15 oz) can diced tomatoes
- 1 cup low•sodium chicken or vegetable broth
- Salt and pepper to taste
- Toppings: shredded cheese, diced avocado, chopped cilantro, lime wedges

Instructions:

1. In a large pot or Dutch oven, cook the ground turkey over medium•high heat, breaking it up with a wooden spoon, until browned and cooked through, about 5•7 minutes. Drain any excess fat.

2. Add the olive oil, onion, garlic, and jalapeños to the pot. Sauté for 2•3 minutes until the vegetables are softened.

3. Stir in the chili powder, cumin, oregano, smoked paprika, and cayenne (if using). Cook for 1 minute to toast the spices.

4. Add the black beans, diced tomatoes, and broth. Bring the mixture to a simmer and let it cook for 15•20 minutes, stirring occasionally, until thickened.

5. Season the chili with salt and pepper to taste.

6. Serve the Spicy Turkey & Black Bean Chili hot, topped with shredded cheese, diced avocado, chopped cilantro, and lime wedges.

Enjoy this hearty and flavorful chili! The combination of lean turkey, black beans, and spices makes it a nutritious and satisfying meal.

107. Roasted Sweet Potato & Quinoa Bowl

Ingredient:

• 2 medium sweet potatoes, peeled and diced into 1•inch cubes
• 2 tbsp olive oil
• 1 tsp ground cumin
• 1/2 tsp chili powder
• Salt and pepper to taste
• 1 cup uncooked quinoa, rinsed
• 2 cups vegetable or chicken broth
• 1 cup baby spinach, chopped
• 1/2 cup canned black beans, drained and rinsed
• 1/4 cup crumbled feta cheese
• 2 tbsp chopped fresh cilantro
• 1 tbsp lime juice

Instructions:

1. Preheat your oven to 400°F (200°C). Line a baking sheet with parchment paper.

2. In a large bowl, toss the diced sweet potatoes with the olive oil, cumin, chili powder, and a pinch of salt and pepper.

3. Spread the seasoned sweet potato cubes in a single layer on the prepared baking sheet. Roast for 20•25 minutes, flipping halfway, until the potatoes are tender and lightly browned.

4. While the sweet potatoes are roasting, cook the quinoa. Bring the quinoa and broth to a boil in a saucepan. Reduce heat, cover, and simmer for 15•20 minutes, until the quinoa is tender and the liquid is absorbed. Fluff with a fork.

5. In a large bowl, combine the roasted sweet potatoes, cooked quinoa, chopped spinach, black beans, crumbled feta, and chopped cilantro.

6. Drizzle the lime juice over the bowl and toss gently to combine.

7. Serve the Roasted Sweet Potato & Quinoa Bowl warm or at room temperature.

This colorful and nutrient•dense bowl makes a great vegetarian or vegan•friendly meal. The combination of roasted sweet potatoes, quinoa, greens, and beans provides a balance of complex carbohydrates, protein, and healthy fats.

108. Teriyaki Chicken Skewers

Ingredient:

- 1 lb boneless, skinless chicken breasts, cut into 1•inch cubes
- 1/2 cup teriyaki sauce (store•bought or homemade)
- 2 tbsp brown sugar
- 1 tbsp rice vinegar
- 1 tsp sesame oil
- 1 tsp grated fresh ginger
- 2 cloves garlic, minced
- 1/4 tsp red pepper flakes (optional)
- Salt and pepper to taste
- Wooden or metal skewers

Instructions:

1. In a medium bowl, whisk together the teriyaki sauce, brown sugar, rice vinegar, sesame oil, grated ginger, minced garlic, and red pepper flakes (if using). Season with a pinch of salt and pepper.

2. Add the cubed chicken to the marinade and toss to coat evenly. Cover and refrigerate for at least 30 minutes, up to 4 hours.

3. Preheat your grill or grill pan to medium•high heat.

4. Thread the marinated chicken cubes onto the skewers, leaving a little space between each piece.

5. Grill the chicken skewers for 2•3 minutes per side, or until the chicken is cooked through and slightly charred.

6. Serve the Teriyaki Chicken Skewers immediately, with any remaining teriyaki sauce drizzled over the top or on the side for dipping.

These Teriyaki Chicken Skewers make a great appetizer or main dish. The sweet and savory teriyaki marinade caramelizes on the grill, creating a delicious flavor. Serve them with steamed rice, a fresh salad, or your favorite grilled vegetables for a complete and satisfying meal.

109. Garlic Herb Roasted Brussels Sprouts

Ingredient:

• 1 lb Brussels sprouts, trimmed and halved
• 2 tbsp olive oil
• 3 cloves garlic, minced
• 1 tsp dried thyme
• 1 tsp dried rosemary
• 1/2 tsp salt
• 1/4 tsp black pepper
• Zest of 1 lemon (optional)
• Chopped fresh parsley for garnish (optional)

Instructions:

1. Preheat your oven to 400°F (200°C). Line a baking sheet with parchment paper or foil.

2. In a large bowl, toss the trimmed and halved Brussels sprouts with the olive oil, minced garlic, dried thyme, dried rosemary, salt, and black pepper until the sprouts are evenly coated.

3. Spread the seasoned Brussels sprouts in a single layer on the prepared baking sheet.

4. Roast the Brussels sprouts in the preheated oven for 20•25 minutes, tossing halfway, until they are tender and lightly browned.

5. Remove the roasted Brussels sprouts from the oven and transfer them to a serving bowl.

6. If desired, zest the lemon over the top of the Brussels sprouts and garnish with chopped fresh parsley.

7. Serve the Garlic Herb Roasted Brussels Sprouts hot, as a side dish or part of a larger meal.

These Garlic Herb Roasted Brussels Sprouts are a delicious and easy•to•prepare vegetable side dish. The combination of garlic, herbs, and a touch of lemon zest adds tons of flavor to the roasted Brussels sprouts. Enjoy them as a healthy and flavorful accompaniment to your main course.

110. Mediterranean Veggie Bowl

Ingredient:

- 1 cup cooked quinoa
- 1 cup chopped cucumber
- 1 cup cherry tomatoes, halved
- 1/2 cup diced red onion
- 1/2 cup crumbled feta cheese
- 1/4 cup kalamata olives, sliced
- 2 tbsp chopped fresh parsley
- 2 tbsp olive oil
- 1 tbsp red wine vinegar
- 1 tsp dried oregano
- 1/4 tsp salt
- 1/4 tsp black pepper

Instructions:

1. In a large bowl, combine the cooked quinoa, chopped cucumber, cherry tomatoes, diced red onion, crumbled feta cheese, and sliced kalamata olives.

2. In a small bowl, whisk together the olive oil, red wine vinegar, dried oregano, salt, and black pepper.

3. Pour the dressing over the vegetable and quinoa mixture and toss gently to coat everything evenly.

4. Sprinkle the chopped fresh parsley over the top of the Mediterranean Veggie Bowl.

5. Serve the bowl immediately, or refrigerate for up to 3 days.

This Mediterranean Veggie Bowl is a nutritious and flavorful vegetarian dish. The combination of quinoa, fresh vegetables, tangy feta, and briny olives creates a delicious and satisfying meal. You can enjoy it as a main dish or as a side.

Feel free to customize the ingredients based on your preferences. For example, you could add chickpeas, roasted red peppers, or grilled zucchini. This bowl is a great way to incorporate more plant·based foods into your diet.

111. Balsamic Glazed Steak

Ingredient:

- 1 lb flank steak or skirt steak
- 2 tbsp olive oil
- 1/4 cup balsamic vinegar
- 2 tbsp brown sugar
- 2 cloves garlic, minced
- 1 tsp Dijon mustard
- 1/2 tsp dried thyme
- 1/4 tsp red pepper flakes (optional)
- Salt and pepper to taste

Instructions:

1. In a shallow baking dish or resealable plastic bag, combine the olive oil, balsamic vinegar, brown sugar, garlic, Dijon mustard, thyme, and red pepper flakes (if using). Season with salt and pepper.

2. Add the steak to the marinade and turn to coat both sides. Cover and refrigerate for at least 30 minutes, up to 4 hours.

3. Preheat your grill or grill pan to medium·high heat.

4. Remove the steak from the marinade and discard any remaining marinade.

5. Grill the steak for 3·5 minutes per side, or until it reaches your desired level of doneness. For medium·rare, the internal temperature should be around 130·135°F (54·57°C).

6. Transfer the grilled steak to a cutting board and let it rest for 5·10 minutes before slicing against the grain into thin strips.

7. Serve the Balsamic Glazed Steak immediately, drizzling any accumulated juices from the cutting board over the top.

This balsamic·glazed steak is full of flavor and makes for a delicious and easy·to·prepare main dish. The sweet and tangy marinade caramelizes on the grill, creating a beautiful glaze on the steak. Enjoy it with roasted vegetables, mashed potatoes, or a fresh salad.

112. Greek Yogurt & Berry Parfait

Ingredient:

• 2 cups plain Greek yogurt
• 2 tbsp honey (or maple syrup)
• 1 tsp vanilla extract
• 1 cup fresh or frozen mixed berries (such as blueberries, raspberries, and blackberries)
• 1/2 cup granola (homemade or store•bought)

Instructions:

1. In a medium bowl, mix together the Greek yogurt, honey (or maple syrup), and vanilla extract until well combined.

2. In parfait glasses or small bowls, layer the yogurt mixture and the mixed berries, starting and ending with the yogurt.

3. Top each parfait with a sprinkling of granola.

4. Refrigerate the parfaits for at least 30 minutes before serving to allow the flavors to meld.

5. Serve the Greek Yogurt & Berry Parfaits chilled.

Optional Variations:
• Use different types of berries or fruit, such as sliced strawberries, diced mango, or chopped pineapple.
• Sprinkle toasted nuts, shredded coconut, or chia seeds on top of the parfaits.
• Substitute low•fat or non•fat Greek yogurt to reduce the calorie and fat content.
• Use honey•flavored or vanilla•flavored Greek yogurt to add more sweetness.

This Greek Yogurt & Berry Parfait makes a delicious and healthy breakfast, snack, or dessert. The creamy yogurt, sweet berries, and crunchy granola create a satisfying and nutritious treat. Enjoy!

113. Spicy Chickpea & Veggie Bowl

Ingredient:

- 1 (15 oz) can chickpeas, drained and rinsed
- 2 tbsp olive oil
- 1 tsp chili powder
- 1/2 tsp cumin
- 1/4 tsp cayenne pepper (or to taste)
- Salt and pepper to taste
- 1 cup cooked quinoa
- 1 cup chopped kale
- 1 cup diced bell pepper
- 1/2 cup diced red onion
- 1/4 cup crumbled feta cheese
- 2 tbsp chopped fresh cilantro
- 1 tbsp lime juice

Instructions:

1. Preheat your oven to 400°F (200°C). Line a baking sheet with parchment paper.

2. In a bowl, toss the drained and rinsed chickpeas with the olive oil, chili powder, cumin, cayenne pepper, and a pinch of salt and pepper.

3. Spread the seasoned chickpeas in a single layer on the prepared baking sheet. Roast for 15•20 minutes, stirring halfway, until crispy.

4. In a large bowl, combine the cooked quinoa, chopped kale, diced bell pepper, diced red onion, crumbled feta cheese, and chopped cilantro.

5. Add the roasted spicy chickpeas to the bowl and drizzle with the lime juice. Toss everything together gently.

6. Serve the Spicy Chickpea & Veggie Bowl warm or at room temperature.

This colorful and flavorful bowl is packed with plant•based protein, fiber, and nutrients. The roasted spicy chickpeas add a delicious crunch, while the quinoa, vegetables, and feta provide a variety of textures and flavors. Adjust the amount of cayenne pepper to your desired level of spiciness.

This dish makes a great vegetarian or vegan•friendly main meal, but you can also serve it as a side. Enjoy!

114. Maple Cinnamon Roasted Carrots

Ingredient:

- 1 lb carrots, peeled and cut into 1·inch pieces
- 2 tbsp olive oil
- 2 tbsp pure maple syrup
- 1 tsp ground cinnamon
- 1/4 tsp salt
- 1/4 tsp black pepper

Instructions:

1. Preheat your oven to 400°F (200°C). Line a baking sheet with parchment paper.

2. In a large bowl, toss the peeled and cut carrots with the olive oil, maple syrup, cinnamon, salt, and black pepper until the carrots are evenly coated.

3. Spread the seasoned carrots in a single layer on the prepared baking sheet.

4. Roast the carrots in the preheated oven for 20·25 minutes, tossing halfway, until they are tender and lightly caramelized.

5. Remove the roasted carrots from the oven and transfer them to a serving dish.

6. Serve the Maple Cinnamon Roasted Carrots warm, as a side dish or snack.

These Maple Cinnamon Roasted Carrots are a simple and delicious way to prepare this nutritious vegetable. The maple syrup and cinnamon create a sweet and aromatic glaze that caramelizes on the carrots as they roast.

The combination of flavors makes these carrots a perfect accompaniment to roasted meats, grilled fish, or as part of a larger vegetable·focused meal. You can also enjoy them on their own as a healthy snack.

Feel free to adjust the amount of maple syrup or cinnamon to suit your taste preferences. This recipe is easy to scale up or down depending on the number of servings you need.

115. Lemon Herb Grilled Shrimp

Ingredient:

- 1 lb large shrimp, peeled and deveined
- 2 tbsp olive oil
- 2 tbsp freshly squeezed lemon juice
- 2 tsp lemon zest
- 2 cloves garlic, minced
- 1 tbsp chopped fresh parsley
- 1 tbsp chopped fresh basil
- 1/2 tsp dried oregano
- 1/4 tsp red pepper flakes (optional)
- Salt and pepper to taste

Instructions:

1. In a large bowl, combine the shrimp, olive oil, lemon juice, lemon zest, minced garlic, chopped parsley, chopped basil, dried oregano, and red pepper flakes (if using). Season with salt and pepper.

2. Toss the shrimp to coat them evenly with the marinade. Cover and refrigerate for 30 minutes to 1 hour.

3. Preheat your grill or grill pan to medium•high heat.

4. Thread the marinated shrimp onto metal or wooden skewers, leaving a little space between each shrimp.

5. Grill the shrimp skewers for 2•3 minutes per side, or until the shrimp are opaque and cooked through.

6. Serve the Lemon Herb Grilled Shrimp immediately, garnished with additional chopped parsley or basil if desired.

These Lemon Herb Grilled Shrimp make a delicious and easy•to•prepare main dish or appetizer. The bright, fresh flavors of the lemon, herbs, and garlic complement the sweet, juicy shrimp perfectly. Serve them with grilled vegetables, over a salad, or alongside rice or pasta for a complete meal.

116. Mushroom and Quinoa Skillet

Ingredient:

- 1 cup uncooked quinoa, rinsed
- 2 cups vegetable or chicken broth
- 2 tbsp olive oil
- 8 oz cremini or button mushrooms, sliced
- 1 small onion, diced
- 3 cloves garlic, minced
- 1 tsp dried thyme
- 1/2 tsp dried oregano
- 1/4 tsp red pepper flakes (optional)
- Salt and pepper to taste
- 2 cups baby spinach, chopped
- 1/4 cup grated Parmesan cheese (optional)
- Chopped fresh parsley for garnish

Instructions:

1. In a medium saucepan, combine the rinsed quinoa and broth. Bring to a boil, then reduce heat, cover, and simmer for 15•20 minutes, until the quinoa is tender and the liquid is absorbed. Fluff with a fork.

2. In a large skillet, heat the olive oil over medium•high heat. Add the sliced mushrooms and cook for 5•7 minutes, until they are browned and tender.

3. Add the diced onion and minced garlic to the skillet. Sauté for 2•3 minutes until the onion is translucent.

4. Stir in the cooked quinoa, dried thyme, dried oregano, and red pepper flakes (if using). Season with salt and pepper to taste.

5. Add the chopped baby spinach to the skillet and cook for 1•2 minutes, just until the spinach is wilted.

6. Remove the skillet from heat and stir in the grated Parmesan cheese, if using. Serve the Mushroom and Quinoa Skillet warm, garnished with chopped fresh parsley.

This one•pan Mushroom and Quinoa Skillet is a nutritious and flavorful vegetarian dish. The combination of earthy mushrooms, fluffy quinoa, and nutrient•rich spinach makes it a satisfying and wholesome meal. Adjust the seasonings to your taste preferences.

117. Cabbage and Tofu Stir·Fry

Ingredient:

• 1 block (14 oz) extra·firm tofu, pressed and cubed
• 2 tbsp sesame oil, divided
• 3 cups shredded green cabbage
• 1 cup shredded carrots
• 1 red bell pepper, thinly sliced
• 3 cloves garlic, minced
• 1 tbsp grated fresh ginger
• 2 tbsp low·sodium soy sauce
• 1 tbsp rice vinegar
• 1 tsp sesame seeds
• Salt and pepper to taste
• Chopped green onions for garnish (optional)

Instructions:

1. In a large skillet or wok, heat 1 tbsp of the sesame oil over medium·high heat. Add the cubed tofu and cook, stirring occasionally, until lightly browned on all sides, about 5·7 minutes. Transfer the tofu to a plate and set aside.

2. In the same skillet, heat the remaining 1 tbsp of sesame oil over medium·high heat. Add the shredded cabbage, carrots, and sliced bell pepper. Stir·fry for 3·4 minutes, until the vegetables are starting to soften.

3. Add the minced garlic and grated ginger to the skillet. Cook for 1 minute, until fragrant.

4. Return the cooked tofu to the skillet. Pour in the soy sauce and rice vinegar. Toss everything together and cook for 2·3 minutes more, until the vegetables are tender·crisp.

5. Remove the Cabbage and Tofu Stir·Fry from heat and stir in the sesame seeds. Season with salt and pepper to taste.

6. Serve the stir·fry hot, garnished with chopped green onions if desired. Enjoy!

This Cabbage and Tofu Stir·Fry is a quick, healthy, and flavorful vegetarian dish. The combination of crunchy cabbage, carrots, bell pepper, and crispy tofu, all tossed in a savory soy·ginger sauce, makes for a delicious and satisfying meal.

*Congratulations on completing your journey through the **Fit Men Cookbook!** We hope this collection of over 110 quick and healthy recipes has empowered you to eat well, feel energized, and conquer your busy days with ease.*

This cookbook was crafted with the modern man in mind, recognizing the challenges of maintaining a healthy lifestyle amidst a hectic schedule. Whether you're hitting the gym, powering through a workday, or simply striving to eat better, these recipes are designed to support your goals without sacrificing flavor or convenience.

As you continue to explore the recipes and techniques shared in this book, remember that healthy eating is not just about fueling your body—it's about enjoying the process and nurturing your well-being. From vibrant breakfasts to hearty dinners, each dish has been thoughtfully selected to provide balanced nutrition and culinary satisfaction.

*Thank you for allowing the **Fit Men Cookbook** to be a part of your journey towards better health and vitality. May these recipes continue to inspire you to prioritize your wellness and make delicious, nutritious choices in every meal.*

Here's to living fit, eating well, and embracing the joy of cooking for a healthier, happier you!

116. Mushroom and Quinoa Skillet

Ingredient:

- 1 cup uncooked quinoa, rinsed
- 2 cups vegetable or chicken broth
- 2 tbsp olive oil
- 8 oz cremini or button mushrooms, sliced
- 1 small onion, diced
- 3 cloves garlic, minced
- 1 tsp dried thyme
- 1/2 tsp dried oregano
- 1/4 tsp red pepper flakes (optional)
- Salt and pepper to taste
- 2 cups baby spinach, chopped
- 1/4 cup grated Parmesan cheese (optional)
- Chopped fresh parsley for garnish

Instructions:

1. In a medium saucepan, combine the rinsed quinoa and broth. Bring to a boil, then reduce heat, cover, and simmer for 15•20 minutes, until the quinoa is tender and the liquid is absorbed. Fluff with a fork.

2. In a large skillet, heat the olive oil over medium•high heat. Add the sliced mushrooms and cook for 5•7 minutes, until they are browned and tender.

3. Add the diced onion and minced garlic to the skillet. Sauté for 2•3 minutes until the onion is translucent.

4. Stir in the cooked quinoa, dried thyme, dried oregano, and red pepper flakes (if using). Season with salt and pepper to taste.

5. Add the chopped baby spinach to the skillet and cook for 1•2 minutes, just until the spinach is wilted.

6. Remove the skillet from heat and stir in the grated Parmesan cheese, if using. Serve the Mushroom and Quinoa Skillet warm, garnished with chopped fresh parsley.

This one•pan Mushroom and Quinoa Skillet is a nutritious and flavorful vegetarian dish. The combination of earthy mushrooms, fluffy quinoa, and nutrient•rich spinach makes it a satisfying and wholesome meal. Adjust the seasonings to your taste preferences.

117. Cabbage and Tofu Stir·Fry

Ingredient:

- 1 block (14 oz) extra·firm tofu, pressed and cubed
- 2 tbsp sesame oil, divided
- 3 cups shredded green cabbage
- 1 cup shredded carrots
- 1 red bell pepper, thinly sliced
- 3 cloves garlic, minced
- 1 tbsp grated fresh ginger
- 2 tbsp low·sodium soy sauce
- 1 tbsp rice vinegar
- 1 tsp sesame seeds
- Salt and pepper to taste
- Chopped green onions for garnish (optional)

Instructions:

1. In a large skillet or wok, heat 1 tbsp of the sesame oil over medium·high heat. Add the cubed tofu and cook, stirring occasionally, until lightly browned on all sides, about 5·7 minutes. Transfer the tofu to a plate and set aside.

2. In the same skillet, heat the remaining 1 tbsp of sesame oil over medium·high heat. Add the shredded cabbage, carrots, and sliced bell pepper. Stir·fry for 3·4 minutes, until the vegetables are starting to soften.

3. Add the minced garlic and grated ginger to the skillet. Cook for 1 minute, until fragrant.

4. Return the cooked tofu to the skillet. Pour in the soy sauce and rice vinegar. Toss everything together and cook for 2·3 minutes more, until the vegetables are tender·crisp.

5. Remove the Cabbage and Tofu Stir·Fry from heat and stir in the sesame seeds. Season with salt and pepper to taste.

6. Serve the stir·fry hot, garnished with chopped green onions if desired. Enjoy!

This Cabbage and Tofu Stir·Fry is a quick, healthy, and flavorful vegetarian dish. The combination of crunchy cabbage, carrots, bell pepper, and crispy tofu, all tossed in a savory soy·ginger sauce, makes for a delicious and satisfying meal.

*Congratulations on completing your journey through the **Fit Men Cookbook!** We hope this collection of over 110 quick and healthy recipes has empowered you to eat well, feel energized, and conquer your busy days with ease.*

This cookbook was crafted with the modern man in mind, recognizing the challenges of maintaining a healthy lifestyle amidst a hectic schedule. Whether you're hitting the gym, powering through a workday, or simply striving to eat better, these recipes are designed to support your goals without sacrificing flavor or convenience.

As you continue to explore the recipes and techniques shared in this book, remember that healthy eating is not just about fueling your body—it's about enjoying the process and nurturing your well-being. From vibrant breakfasts to hearty dinners, each dish has been thoughtfully selected to provide balanced nutrition and culinary satisfaction.

*Thank you for allowing the **Fit Men Cookbook** to be a part of your journey towards better health and vitality. May these recipes continue to inspire you to prioritize your wellness and make delicious, nutritious choices in every meal.*

Here's to living fit, eating well, and embracing the joy of cooking for a healthier, happier you!